Tai Chi and Qigong for Health:
A Framework for Understanding

Hand of the Wind Taijiquan

Introduction.

This book is intended to provide a framework for understanding of some of the theory behind Tai Chi and Qigong for health in order to enable students of Hand of the Wind Taijiquan to get more benefit from their practice of Tai Chi and Qigong. This is a book of theory and does not teach the Tai Chi Forms or Qigong exercises – see our other publications for training guides.

This book represents an accumulation of knowledge and insights that have been developed over more than a quarter of a century spent training in the Lee Family Internal Arts of Tai Chi and Qigong alongside my personal study of the correlations between Qigong and Chinese Medicine. Wherever possible, throughout this book I have tried to present the theory behind Tai Chi and Qigong without using technical Chinese 'jargon' – there often seems to be a tradition of using language as a way of concealing information within the Chinese martial arts and this is something I do not wish to do.

There are many interpretations of Tai Chi Theory (probably as many as there are instructors!) and so you may find things in this book that you disagree with or contradict what you have been taught by other Tai Chi Instructors. What I have tried to do with this book is to provide information that is accessible to all students and that is of practical use within the context of Tai Chi and Qigong training for health rather than martial purposes.

How much of the information in this book you choose to implement into your own training is of course entirely up to you! Section One of this volume covers aspects of Chinese Medicine and how it relates to our training. Section Two covers more practical/physical aspects to be aware of when practicing.

Tai Chi and Qigong for Health: A Framework for Understanding.

Hand of the Wind Taijiquan.

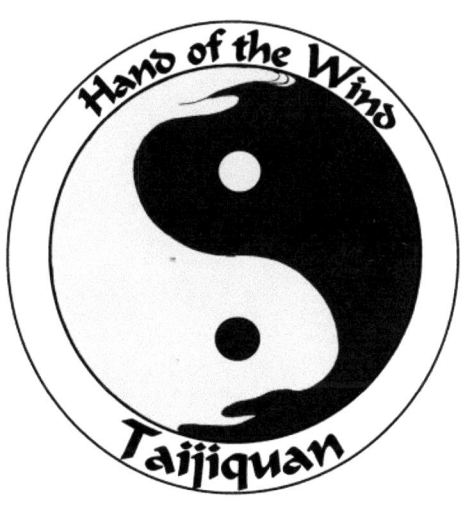

Conrad Robinson

Contents:

Chapter One.

What are Tai Chi and Qigong?

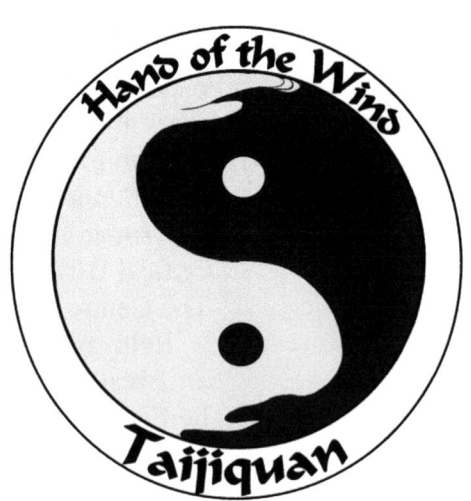

The question of what are Tai Chi and Qigong is the first question a student usually asks and is one of the hardest to answer.

A definition of Tai Chi Ch'uan (or Taijiquan – there are various ways in which Chinese can be written in English) could simply be: An Internal Chinese Martial Art based upon the principles of Yin and Yang. However, this just raises more questions, Internal? Yin and Yang? 'Martial Art – I thought it was a health exercise?'

So first, let us address the Internal Martial Art bit. Tai Chi Ch'uan (usually just referred to as Tai Chi) originated as a martial art and as it developed it also became known for its benefits to health. The health benefits were originally a side-effect of the martial art training but in the modern world the majority of people train Tai Chi just for the health benefits and have no interest in the martial aspects. This is fine – Tai Chi is an excellent health exercise system suitable for people of all ages and can be practiced by people with a wide variety of health conditions. An interest in the martial side of the art is completely optional! Having said that, students at Hand of the Wind classes will be used to at least seeing martial aspects of movements demonstrated, as it does help to fully understand the movements.

When we describe Tai Chi as an Internal martial art (in simple terms) we mean that it is a relaxed system where power is generated internally through an understanding of Qigong and not by using muscular tension as in the so-called 'External' martial arts. External martial arts include Karate, Taekwondo, Jujitsu, Kung Fu and many others. The main three Chinese martial arts, considered as Internal are: Taijiquan, Baguazhuang and Xing Yi Quan.

Kung Fu can be considered as somewhat problematical in the list of External martial arts as Chee Soo taught the martial aspects of Lee Family Taijiquan under the banner of Feng Shou Kung Fu - this was essentially a commercial decision by Chee Soo in order to attract students to the Arts at a time when the term Kung Fu was becoming familiar to Westerners, largely due to the films of Bruce Lee. It is of interest to note that Kung Fu literally translates as 'hard work'.

If we break down the name of Tai Chi Ch'uan, the Ch'uan part is what defines the art as a martial art and is often translated as 'fist' so Tai Chi Ch'uan could be said to be 'Fist of Tai Chi'. Tai Chi is often translated as something like 'The Supreme Ultimate' or 'The Great Ridgepole' but for simplicity's sake can just be considered as the correct name of the symbol that most people in the West would call 'a Yin and Yang'.

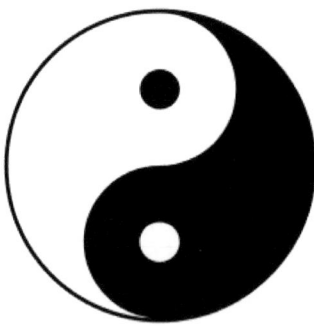

We then come to the definition of Taijiquan as Yin and Yang Fist. So next, we need to consider the question of 'what is Yin and Yang'?

To put it into its simplest terms for a practical understanding which is useful to us in our Tai Chi and Qigong training, think of Yin as contraction and inward movement and think of Yang as expansion and outward movement. We shall explore this more in the later chapter on Yin and Yang.

Having arrived at some kind of definition for what the term Tai Chi Ch'uan means, we need to consider what that actually translates to in practical terms and how it differs (if indeed it does) from Qigong. Therefore, we now need to examine the question of 'what is Qigong?'

Qigong really just means 'to work with Qi' but in order to understand that, we need to consider what we mean by Qi. Again, this is a very difficult question to answer – if you were to ask a native Chinese speaker to translate the word, Qi, they would probably give the English word 'breath'. This seems a very dissatisfying definition and doesn't explain things like Acupuncture, Channels and all the other aspects of Qi that we get used to in our training of Qigong. It becomes a little better if you consider the wider and deeper implications of the word, 'breath' and what it means for life and our existence.

Often you will find people use the term 'Energy' to describe Qi and again this can be problematical – especially to anyone trained in the Sciences where energy has a very specific meaning. So, where does that leave us in our search for a translation of Qi? Qi is a concept which is very firmly embedded within Chinese culture and within the Chinese Medical systems – it does require a different way of looking at the universe which brings us on to the idea of Taoism, discussed more in Chapter Two. The most practical approach is to just think of Qi as Qi and not try to give it an English name.

For the purposes of our Tai Chi and Qigong training, Qi can be considered to be ubiquitous and a fundamental part of our universe. It flows through our bodies (and everything else) and is an essential part of our existence. From a Chinese Medical perspective, Qi flows through specific pathways within our bodies and the surface manifestations of these pathways are the Channels used by Acupuncturists and other therapists. Qi is also stored in so-called 'special vessels' and manifests around the surface of the body as 'defensive' Qi.

An important characteristic of Qi is that it can be guided and controlled (to a certain extent at least) by our minds. So, when we practice Qigong, we use physical movement to emphasize the flow along particular Channels along with mental focus to guide our Qi.

Some Qigong practice involves specific exercises (often with directed breathing) such as the Taoyin and Kaimen exercises taught within the Lee Family Arts. Some Qigong involves more meditative practice, as in Standing Qigong. Practice of the Tai Chi Forms is also a type of Qigong training and it is this aspect which makes Tai Chi such an excellent exercise for health.

It is also important to note that Qigong is also used in martial arts training for purposes of inflicting and resisting damage, but these types of Qigong are quite distinct from the health Qigong practices that are normally taught within Hand of the Wind Tai Chi and Qigong classes.

To return to our question of 'What are Tai Chi and Qigong?', we can now begin to appreciate that there is no simple answer. For practical purposes, a definition of 'An exercise system which helps to regulate and balance the flow of Qi throughout our bodies and therefore benefit our health' is probably as useful as any for the majority of students who practice Tai Chi and Qigong for health purposes.

Chapter Two.

Tai Chi and Taoism.

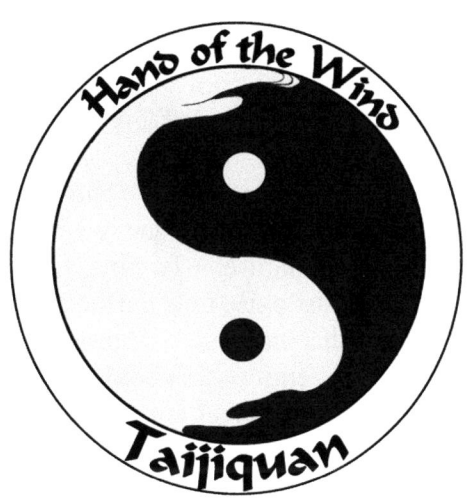

Tai Chi Ch'uan was developed by Taoists within China, so we need to consider what Taoism (pronounced more like D-Ow-Ism) is and how it impacts upon our understanding of the Arts.

Firstly, it is important to point out that Taoism is a philosophy and not a religion as this often causes confusion. It is perfectly possible to consider yourself Taoist and Atheist or Taoist and Catholic, or to combine any other faith system with Taoist philosophy. Often the confusion comes about as people sometimes refer to followers of ancient, traditional spiritual beliefs and religions within China as Taoists and followers of Chan Buddhism or Zen Buddhism can also sometimes be referred to as Taoists. Taoism in itself does not imply the existence, or absence, of any form of Deity or other spiritual power.

The 'Tao' is usually defined as 'The Way' or simply as 'Nature' in the sense that to pursue your Tao is to follow 'your' way or 'your' nature. To find happiness within a Taoist philosophy is to exist in a harmonious way with the Tao or 'nature' of the universe. A thorough discussion of Taoism is beyond the remit of this book but for those who are interested, there are many excellent publications available on the subject. If you want a simple, light hearted guide to understanding the basic principles of Taoism, you might want to consider 'The Tao of Pooh' by Benjamin Hoff.

Lao Tzu's 'Tao Te Ching' is often described as the essential text on Taoism and Chuang Tzu and Lieh Tzu's texts are also well worth looking at if you are interested in gaining an insight into the Chinese thinking around Taoism.

For the purposes of improving our understanding and practice of Tai Chi and Qigong, it is not essential for any student to embrace a Taoist philosophy. It is enough to understand that the origins of the Arts come from a Taoist background.

From a historical perspective, the ruling class in China has generally followed a more Confucianist philosophy rather than Taoist. This led to Taoist Chinese people often being persecuted and helps to explain why Taoist martial arts such as Tai Chi Ch'uan were often practiced in secret and kept hidden within family systems.

Taoism impacts upon our practice of Tai Chi and Qigong mostly in the way that it encourages us to stay relaxed and not force things. Within our training, we look for the relaxation within the movement and posture and this enables us to move in accordance with the principle of the Tao.

Modern sports psychologists often refer to a 'flow state' where the body just seems to work the way it should and things almost become effortless – this is what we mean by moving in accordance with the principle. This is very much at the heart of Tai Chi Ch'uan and is one of the key benefits of our training. We have a system available to us which is designed to help us enter and maintain this 'flow state' and to then apply it to every aspect of our lives.

When we 'move in accordance with the principle' our movements are relaxed and not forced. In our Tai Chi we constantly strive to move with the minimum amount of effort and to not over-stretch ourselves (both physically and psychologically/philosophically). We also focus inwards within our training and get to know ourselves better which helps us find our 'Way' in the world. When we know our own selves better. we can be more confident in the things we do and can become more relaxed and accepting mentally as well as physically – remember in Tai Chi and Qigong there is no distinction between Body and Mind.

Taoism helps us to understand that 'doing' Tai Chi is not just about how we move when we are actively training but is about how it impacts our entire lives. Within a Taoist philosophy, there is an acceptance of the ideas of balance and cycles within the Universe and this informs how we can live our lives in more harmonious ways. The balance between Yin and Yang within our movements in the Tai Chi Forms is achieved through an awareness of how each aspect of our movement cycles through increasing Yin/decreasing Yang and increasing Yang/decreasing Yin (more on this in the next chapter!).

A key thing we should take from Taoism is that how we live our lives matters and that this includes every aspect of our lives. There has been some discussion over recent years about how to refer to people who train in Tai Chi and some people use the term Tai Chi Players. Personally, I do not like this term – I do not 'play' at Tai Chi, I practice Tai Chi. This is not to suggest that there is no sense of 'play' within my Tai Chi – there is a huge amount, especially in the martial! It simply means that I practice Tai Chi by applying it to all aspects of my life, all the time (not always successfully, I am certainly prepared to admit!).

When things feel 'forced', then the way we are doing them is probably not the best way. This does not mean that we do not put effort into things but it does mean that too much effort leads to tension which then makes things harder to achieve. Remember that in Tai Chi (and therefore in life generally) it is better to apply yourself 85% than 100% as you will achieve far more rather than getting tense and burning yourself out. Even professional sports people will admit that when they try too hard, things do not work out as well. Consider the sprinter 'tightening up' in the last 10 metres and being overtaken by the athletes who are still in 'their' running and therefore he or she misses out on a medal.

So, maybe, embrace the principle of the Tao within your training and allow it to cross over into other aspects of your life and this may help you to enjoy even more benefits from your practice.

Chapter Three.

Yin and Yang.

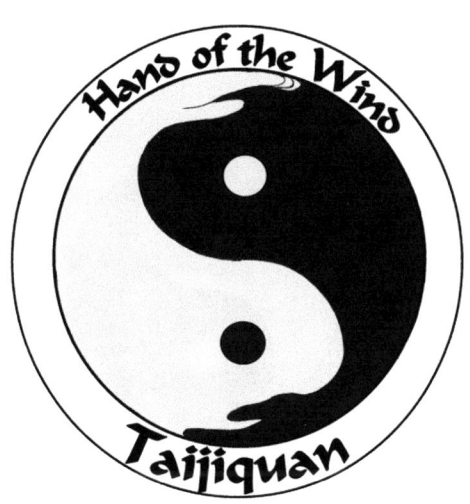

As mentioned previously, in Chapter One, the term Tai Chi describes the symbol that often gets called a 'Yin and Yang' in the West. The fact that our Art is called Tai Chi Ch'uan alerts us to the importance of the concepts of Yin and Yang within our training. So, what are Yin and Yang?

In Chapter One, I stated that for practical purposes within our training the most useful definition is that Yin is contraction and Yang is expansion. This is the aspect of Yin and Yang that I refer to the most when I am teaching Tai Chi and Qigong. However, it is not the only aspect that we should be considering.

The idea of Yin and Yang is at once, very simple and extraordinarily complex. Consider the Tai Chi symbol itself:

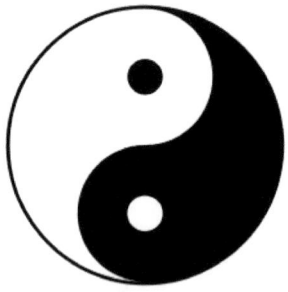

A simple circle, split equally between light and dark, with the light aspect increasing in volume as it moves upwards and the dark aspect increasing as it moves downwards. Where the light aspect is greatest there is an inclusion of the dark aspect at its centre and vice versa. Draw a straight line through the centre on any angle and it will contain an equal amount of light and dark. As one aspect grows the other recedes by an equal amount so that the balance is always maintained.

So, you can see that even from a fairly superficial look this simple symbol contains a large amount of meaning. This is a good indication of some of the complexities around the concepts of Yin and Yang.

An old definition of Yin and Yang was 'the shady and sunny sides of a hill'. So, the 'Yin' side is darker, cooler, damper, etc. And the 'Yang' side is brighter, warmer, drier, etc. These correlations for Yin and Yang can be extended to many other aspects and you will often come across tables of correlations for Yin and Yang.

One of the most important things to remember about Yin and Yang is that neither can exist in isolation – they are both relative terms. Nothing is solely Yin or Yang, but everything can be considered one or the other in relation to something else. If we were to consider what is the most 'Yang' thing we can think of, then most people would probably say the Sun as it is hot, bright, expansive, but compared to a bigger, brighter, hotter star it could be considered to be very Yin.

Often people link gender to Yin and Yang which I consider to be extremely unhelpful. The link between gender (Yang-Male, Yin-Female) is based on the idea that men are more active, more expansive, more aggressive, etc. I would hope that in the modern world we can see that this is nonsensical and indeed the whole concept of binary genders is now being challenged as more of a cultural construct rather than a reflection of reality.

Another often cited correlation which can cause problems with understanding is Yang-hard, Yin-soft. In terms of the physical characteristic of an object this is absolutely fine – it is when people talk about a movement as hard or soft that it can cause issues. Tai Chi is a relaxed form of movement and therefore might be considered soft, some external martial arts seem 'harder' and therefore might be considered Yang to Tai Chi's Yin. But remember that Tai Chi is intended to be in balance between Yin and Yang so thinking about 'hard' and 'soft' is not particularly helpful. An often-used phrase to describe the martial power of Tai Chi

Ch'uan is 'as a steel rod wrapped in velvet'. Anyone who has been on the receiving end of a relaxed, effective strike from a Tai Chi Ch'uan practitioner would not describe it as 'soft'!

Yang as expansive and Yin as contractive is the most practically useful correlation for our training. If you consider any movement of the Tai Chi Form you can quickly determine if the chest is expanding or contracting through the movement. Then consider what that means for the movement of the arms and hands. Always remember that if the chest is expanding, then some other part of the body must be contracting – there is always balance.

As you look at each movement of the Tai Chi Form (or any other exercise) consider which parts of the body are functioning as Yang and which are Yin. Consider front and back, top and bottom, left and right, posture and stance. Examine each of your stances, where are you Yang and where are you Yin within the stance?

Chapter Four.

The Five Transformations.

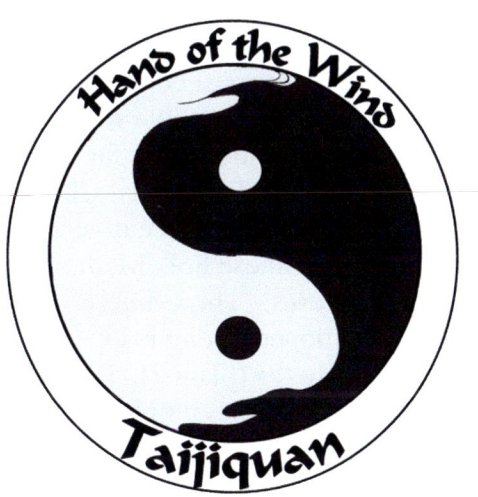

The Five Transformations are more commonly referred to as the Five Elements, but that can cause confusion (especially for anyone familiar with the Greek four elements of Earth, Fire, Water and Air). Within Five Transformation or Five Element theory we do not consider them to be physical elements that mix together to make up the physical things of the Universe. Rather, the Five Elements are phases within the cycle of Yin to Yang to Yin, etc. and this is why it is probably better to refer to them as the Five Transformations.

The Five Transformations are: Fire, Earth, Metal, Water and Tree. Note that Tree is often referred to as Wood, but the idea of a living Tree is a more useful concept than that of dead wood. Metal has at times also been known as Gold or Mountain but Metal is the most commonly used term today.

Within Chinese Medicine, Five Element Theory is used as a simplification of the wider, more far-reaching Traditional Chinese Medicine theory. Traditional Chinese Medicine has become a controversial term in recent years where the media has used it to refer to Chinese Folk Medicine practices which use animal parts as cures. The Chinese herbalism practiced by most TCM practitioners today is exactly that – herbalism which therefore uses herbs (plants!). For the purposes of Tai Chi and Qigong training the simplified medical system of Five Transformations is usually more than sufficient as a framework for understanding how our training can benefit our health.

If we consider each of the Transformations in turn, we can start with Fire (Greater Yang), then Metal (Increasing Yin, Decreasing Yang), to Water (Greater Yin) and then Tree (Increasing Yang, Decreasing Yin). Earth is often placed between Fire and Metal, but can also be considered to be a more balanced state in the centre of the others.

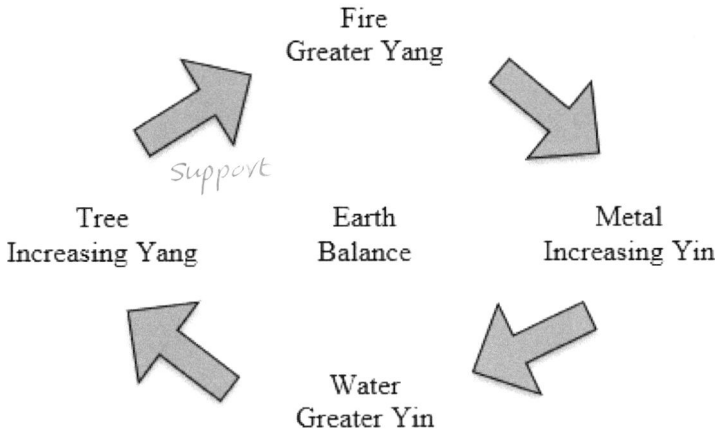

Fig.1 Simplified flow through the Five Transformations.

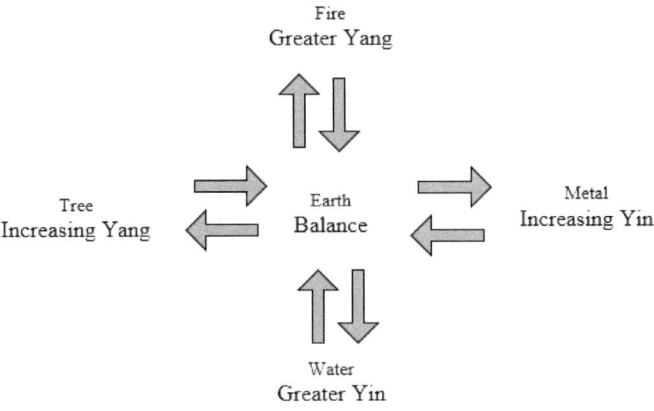

Fig. 2 Alternative view of the flow.

If we look at figure one, we can see that Earth is apparently left out of the flow which does not seem to make sense, so in some older texts you may come across the flow in Figure two. Here Earth creates a balance point between each of the other transformations. In more modern texts you are more likely to come across the flow as shown in Figure 3.

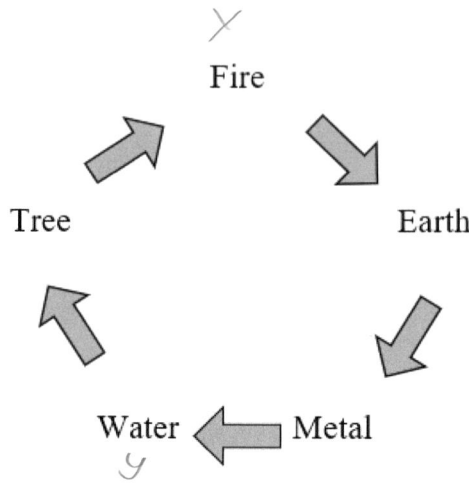

Fig 3. Modern view of the Flow.

   In the clinical usage of Five Transformation Theory the direction of the arrows in Figure one indicates a supportive relationship between the adjacent transformations so Tree can support Fire, etc. This can be useful for a therapist who is aiming to adjust the balance between the Qi within each transformation, and can also be helpful for us when choosing appropriate Qigong exercises to benefit our health. It is important to consult a suitably qualified therapist to seek a diagnosis and advice about how to use Five Transformational Theory to improve health. Figure four shows a pictorial representation of a controlling relationship where water controls fire, etc.

Fire

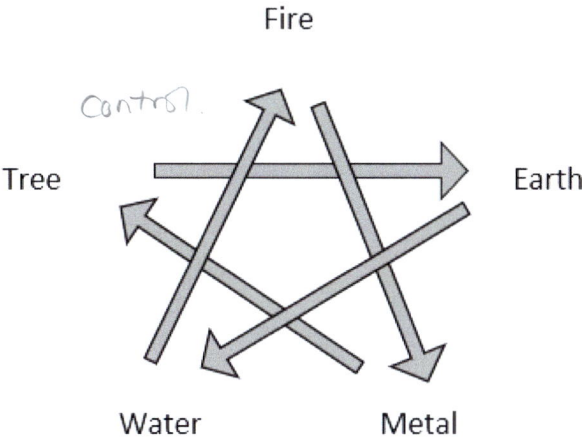

Fig.4 Controlling Cycle of Five Transformations.

If someone is diagnosed as having an excess of Qi within the Channels associated with Fire, then strengthening the Qi in the Water Channels would then have a controlling effect on Fire which would be regarded as beneficial (as shown in Figure four).

If, on the other hand, someone is diagnosed as having a deficit of Qi within the Metal Channels then strengthening the Earth Channels would provide support for the Metal Qi as shown in Figure three.

Remember that you should only apply these principles under the guidance of a properly qualified practitioner of Chinese Medicine who can offer a suitable diagnosis and advice.

Each of the Five Transformations is associated with different aspects of our bodies and therefore governs different aspects of our health. The following table shows some of the associations for each of the Five Transformations.

	Fire	Earth	Metal	Water	Tree
Yin Organ	Heart*	Spleen	Lungs	Kidneys	Liver
Yang Organ	Small Intestine*	Stomach	Large Intestine	Bladder	Gall Bladder
Sensory Organ	Tongue	Lips	Nose	Ears	Eyes
Emotion	Joy	Sympathy	Grief	Fear	Anger
Tissue	Blood Vessels	Muscles	Skin	Bones	Tendons
Season	Summer	Harvest	Autumn	Winter	Spring
* Fire also governs Heart Protector (Yin) and Triple Heater (Yang)					

Fig. 5 Associations of the Five Transformations.

The table in Figure five only shows a few of the Five Transformation associations, focusing on those that are particularly useful within our Tai Chi and Qigong practice.

Each of the Five Transformations is associated with two organ systems and therefore two Qi Channels/Meridians (or four in the case of Fire). These are referred to as the Yin and Yang organs for each Transformation. Generally, the Yin organ is considered to be a 'solid' organ and the Yang organ is a 'hollow' organ, so Yang organs tend to be the intestines or bladders. Fire is unusual as it has two pairs of organs associated with it and in the West more focus is often placed on the Heart and Small Intestine as the concept of Heart Protector and Triple Heater is somewhat alien to us – these are not, after all, physical organs in the sense that we are used to thinking about.

Within Chinese medicine it is common to refer to the Yin organ primarily, so a diagnosis which is linked to the Earth Transformation may be classed as a Spleen diagnosis. Therefore, within Qigong teaching any reference to Heart Qi can also be considered to have relevance for Small Intestine Qi. It is important to remember that Chinese medicine

24

considers the function of the whole organ system and the implications on the body's Qi related to that system rather than focusing purely on the physical organ.

Figure five also shows the seasons that are associated with each of the Five Transformations and again this is where Earth can be somewhat problematical. Each of the other Transformations has a clear season associated with it but Earth is usually associated with either Harvest or Indian Summer to fit in with the modern flow as shown in Figure three where Earth is placed between Fire and Metal. If we look at the older interpretation of the flow as shown in Figure two, we can understand why the older viewpoint was that there was a short 'Earth Season' between each of the other seasons – a time when Qi is in a more settled state between the extremes of each season.

Chapter Five.

The Twelve Channels.

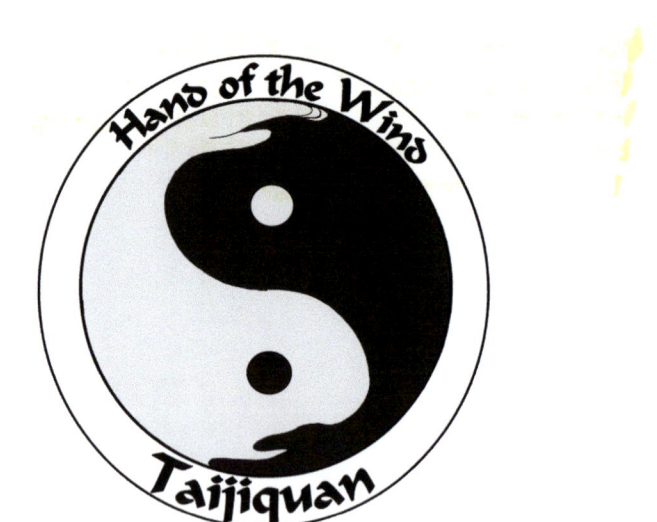

Masunaga channels (japanese channels)

Within this chapter we will look at each pair of Channels associated with each of the Five Transformations. For the purposes of Tai Chi and Qigong training it is not really necessary for every student to have a comprehensive knowledge of the location of every part of each Channel and all of the Acupoints along them. It is, however, very useful to have an awareness of roughly where each Channel flows in the body and to know the start and end points of each Channel. Many people refer to the Channels as 'Meridians' as Chinese Medicine became popular in France before the UK and the French term stuck.

Remember that all of the twelve Channels are each found on the right and left side of the body so that the body is symmetrical. Also, for the purposes of Channel location it is useful to view the body as having the arms raised above the head with the palms facing forwards – this means that the Yin Channels flow upwards and the Yang Channels flow downwards through the body.

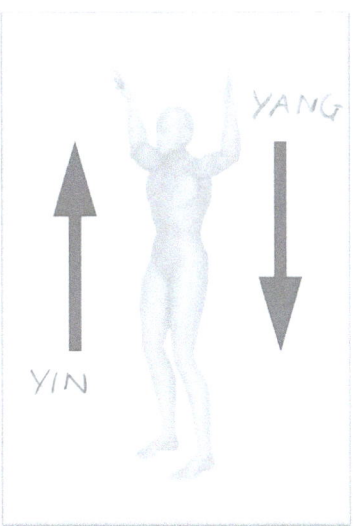

The Fire Channels.

Heart and Small Intestine.

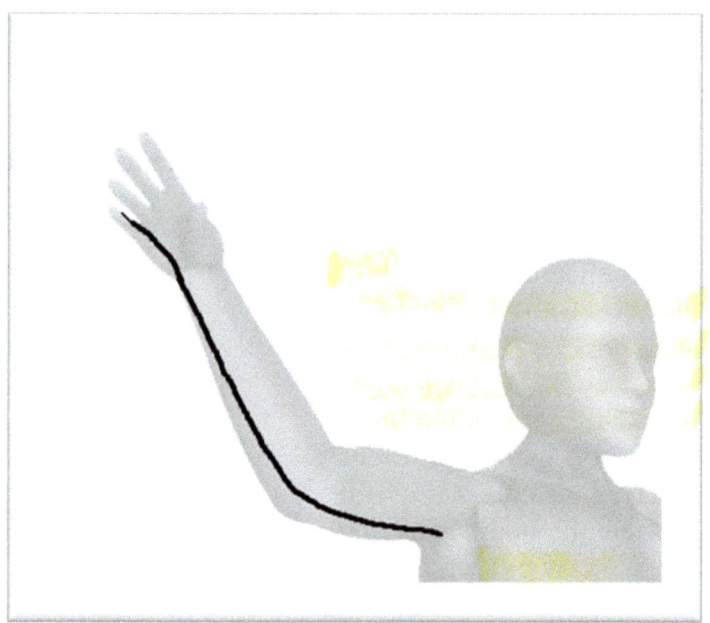

Fig. 7 The Heart Channel

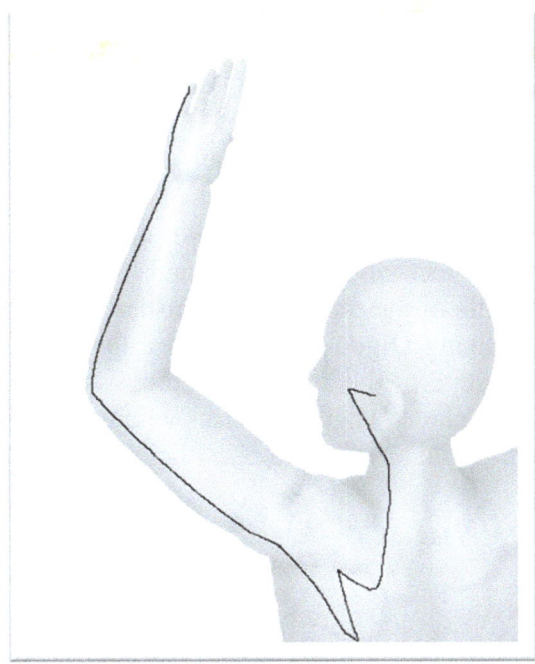

Fig. 8 The Small Intestine Channel.

The Qi within the Heart Channel controls the function of the Heart, in both the physical and metaphorical senses. Heart Qi also governs the blood vessels and the tongue. the sensory organ related to Heart is the tongue and therefore speech and our ability to express ourselves is related to Heart energy. The Small Intestine is associated with assimilation and absorption and therefore with receptivity for both physical food and more metaphorical concepts.

The Heart Channel begins in the centre of the axilla (armpit) and flows upwards along the inner side of the little finger edge of the arm (remembering that the arm is extended upwards above the head in the Chinese anatomical viewpoint). The Heart Channel culminates beside the base of the nail of the little finger (on the side of the nail closest to the ring finger). This means that when the arm is lowered to rest against the body, the Heart Channel is very protected.

The Small Intestine Channel begins beside the base of the nail on the little finger (on the side furthest from the ring finger) and then flows downwards along the little finger edge of the arm (to the rear or outer aspect of the arm). It then 'zigzags' across the shoulder blade before coming up the back of the side of the neck onto the cheek and then passes to in front of the middle of the ear where it finishes.

When practicing Qigong, any exercise that emphasizes the little finger edge of the arm is therefore associated with Heart Qi. This includes many exercises where the hands are raised above the head or raised to chest height in front of the body.

Heart Protector and Triple Heater.

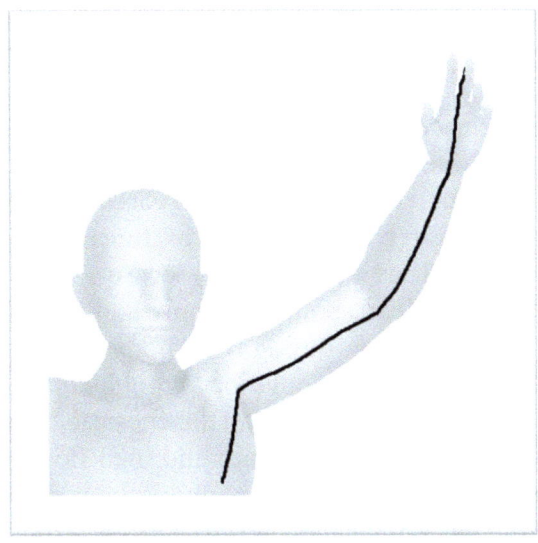

Fig. 9 The Heart Protector Channel. — *p rotect heart*

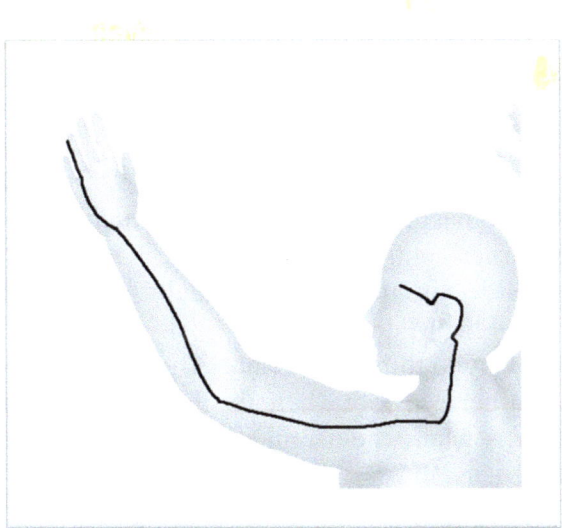

Fig. 10 The Triple Heater Channel.

— *regulate temperature in body.*

31

There are two other Channels associated with the Fire Transformation and they are the Heart Protector and Triple Heater. These can be difficult for people in the West to relate to as they do not have corresponding physical organs in the sense that we are used to.

The Heart Protector is sometimes also known as the Pericardium Channel or sometimes as Circulation/Sex as these can give a clearer idea of some its functions. In the simplest terms the Heart Protector Qi does exactly what it says – it protects the Heart, both physically and emotionally. It also controls blood flow through the body and therefore plays a role in temperature regulation throughout the body. The Heart Protector Channel starts on the chest (to the side of the nipple away from the centre line) and then flows up the centre of the underside of the arm, through the centre of the palm of the hand before finishing beside the nail of the middle finger (towards the thumb edge of the hand).

The Triple Heater Channel (also known as Triple Burner or Triple Warmer) is also involved in regulation of body temperature and in Chinese Medicine is seen to control fluids within the body. Again, in an effort to keep things simple you can think of the Upper Burner as containing the Heart and Lungs (so located above the diaphragm); the Middle Burner contains the Stomach, Spleen and Gall Bladder organs and the Lower Burner contains the Intestines, Kidneys, Bladder (and the Liver despite the Liver physically being within the area covered by the Middle Burner).

A useful way to think of the three Burners is to consider the Middle Burner as a pool where the body heats 'fluids'; the Upper Burner is where the useful 'fluids' are evaporated off and distributed as 'mist' throughout the body; the Lower Burner is like a 'drain' that removes the unwanted fluids. Note that this another area where the simple English term

32

'fluid' does not really convey the ideas as envisaged by Chinese Medicine – don't take things too literally!

The Triple Heater Channel begins next to the nail on the ring finger (on the little finger side), it then flows down the middle of the back of the arm and up the neck to just below the ear. It flows around the back of the ear to just in front of the top of the ear before continuing to finish by the outer edge of the eyebrow.

Within Qigong training, any exercise that emphasizes the Heart Channel will also tend to work the Heart Protector, so arms above the head or to the front – if you adjust the angle of the hands in these positions it can change the emphasis from Heart to Heart Protector. For example, if the hands are raised to chest height, palms forwards in front of the body with the fingers pointing upwards it will emphasize Heart Protector and if the little finger edge is upwards it will emphasize Heart more.

The Earth Channels.

Spleen and Stomach.

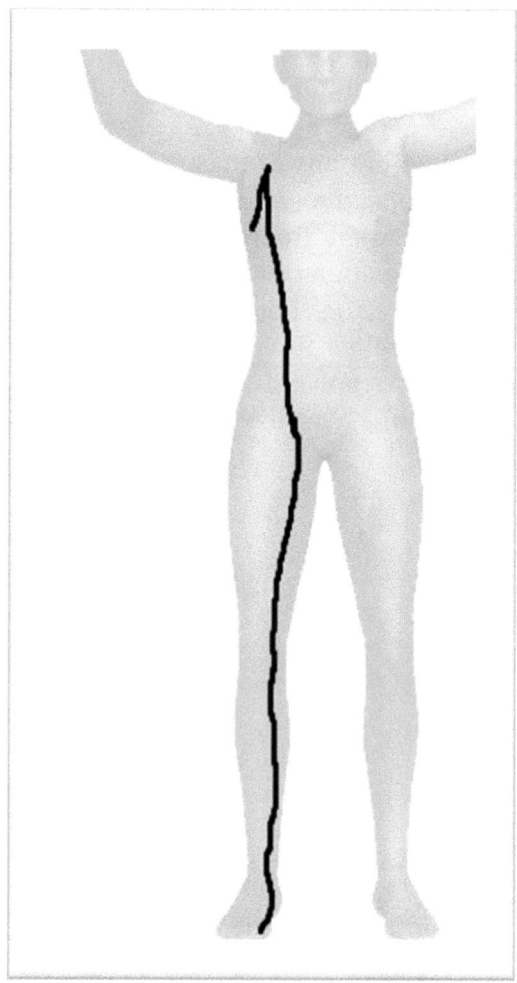

Fig. 11 The Spleen Channel.

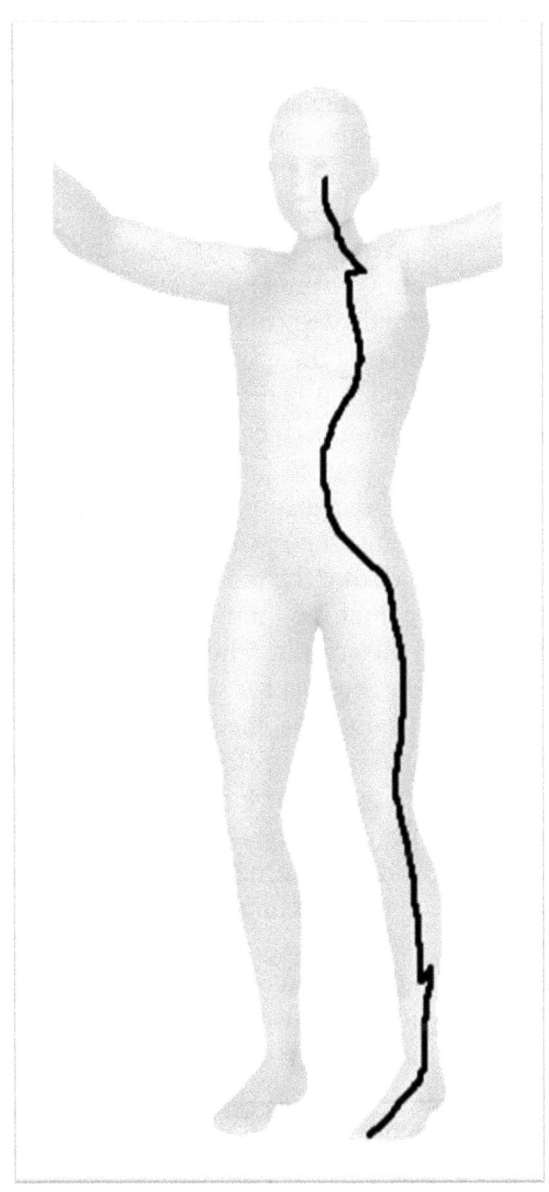

Fig. 12 The Stomach Channel.

Spleen (and therefore Stomach) Qi is associated with digestion, both of foods and ideas and therefore problems with overthinking and worrying are often linked to Spleen Qi. Spleen Qi governs the muscles and is also involved in regulating blood by keeping it within the blood vessels.

The Spleen Channel begins beside the nail of the big toe (on the side furthest from the little toe), passes in front of the medial malleolus (the bony protuberance on the inside of the ankle!) before flowing up the leg (to the front of the inside of the leg). It then flows up past the groin and up the side of the front of the body on a line that takes it towards the shoulder (to the outside of the nipple), then from the front of the shoulder it flows downwards to finish on the side of the ribcage below the front of the armpit (again, for the purposes of our Tai Chi and Qigong training knowledge of the exact location of the end point of the Channel is not really necessary – it is sufficient to know that it culminates on the side of the body below the front of the armpit. There are many excellent resources available on the internet for specific point locations if you are interested in finding the exact location).

The Stomach Channel begins below the centre of the eye (which is why we say that we start eating with our eyes!), it then flows down to the corner of the mouth before continuing down the front of the side of the neck (although there is a branch that splits off at the jawline and extends up to the hairline at the side of the forehead). From the neck, it flows down the front of the shoulder and on a line down through the front of the body (which is unusual for a Yang Channel), through the nipple before moving closer to the centre line as it passes down through the abdomen. From the top of the groin, it flows out to the top of the outside of the thigh (towards the front of the leg) and then down the front of the leg (on the outside 'edge'), past the outside of the front of the knee, across the front of the ankle to finish on the toe next to the big toe (beside the base of the nail towards the little toe side).

Qigong exercises that stretch the front of the legs will be of benefit to Spleen (and therefore Stomach) Qi along with exercises that stretch the side of the body by leaning or twisting the trunk of the body.

The Metal Channels.

Lung and Large Intestine.

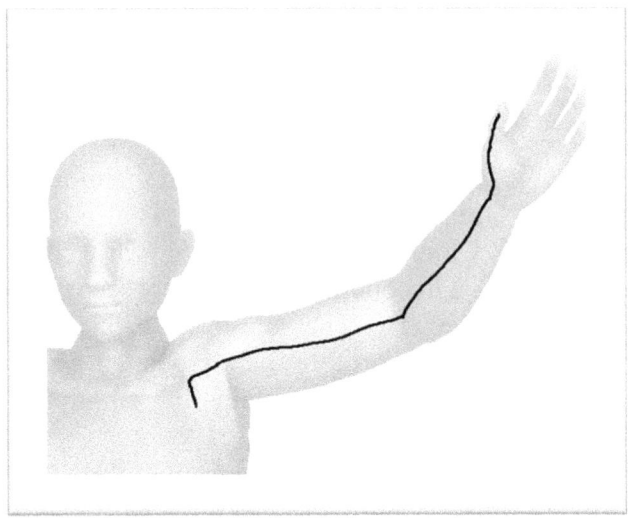

Fig. 13 The Lung Channel.

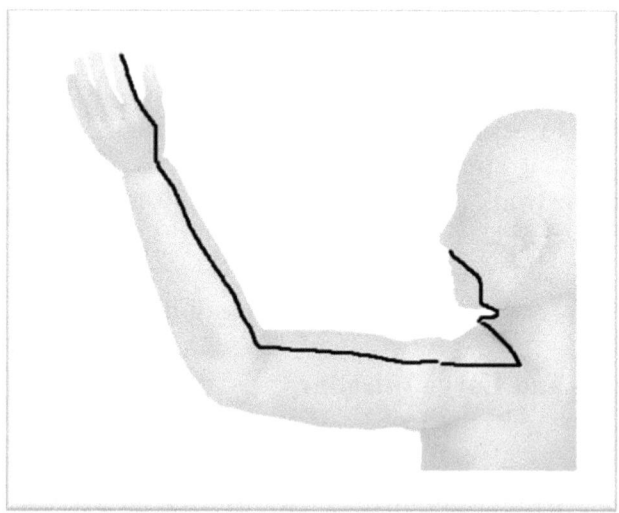

Fig. 14 The Large Intestine Channel.

Lung Qi is associated with breath and therefore with the distribution of Qi throughout the body, it is also responsible for our skin – which helps to explain why correlations between lung and skin conditions are widely recognized even in Western Medicine. The Large Intestine relates to elimination and can therefore be associated with issues relating to 'letting go' – this explains the emotion of grief being associated with Metal.

The Lung Channel begins in the front of the shoulder (in the dip in the muscle below the clavicle) and then flows up the arm along the thumb edge of the inner side of the arm, before finishing beside the base of the thumbnail (on the side farthest from the little finger).

The Large Intestine Channel starts beside the nail of the forefinger and then passes across the muscle between the thumb and forefinger before flowing down the arm along the thumb 'edge' of the outside of the arm. From the shoulder, it flows to the base of the rear of the neck before flowing to the front of the side of the neck and up across the cheek to the bottom of the nose. Uniquely for one of the twelve Channels it then crosses the centre line to finish to the side of the nostril (on the opposite side of the body from where it started – so the Large Intestine Channel that begins on the left forefinger finishes beside the right nostril).

Qigong exercises to benefit Lung Qi are often characterized by movements where the arms are extended to the sides at shoulder height. But be aware that any exercise where the arms are raised may be of benefit to Fire or Metal Channels depending on the position of the hands – try to feel which aspects of the arms are accentuated when the hands are in different positions. For Lung Qigong exercises you are feeling for sensations along the thumb 'edge' of the arm.

The Water Channels.

Kidney and Bladder.

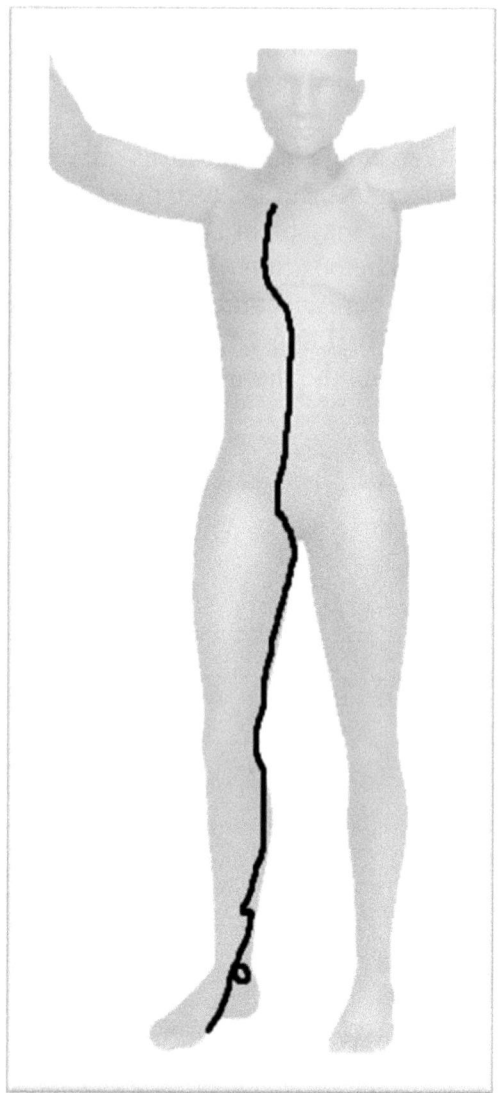

Fig. 15 The Kidney Channel.

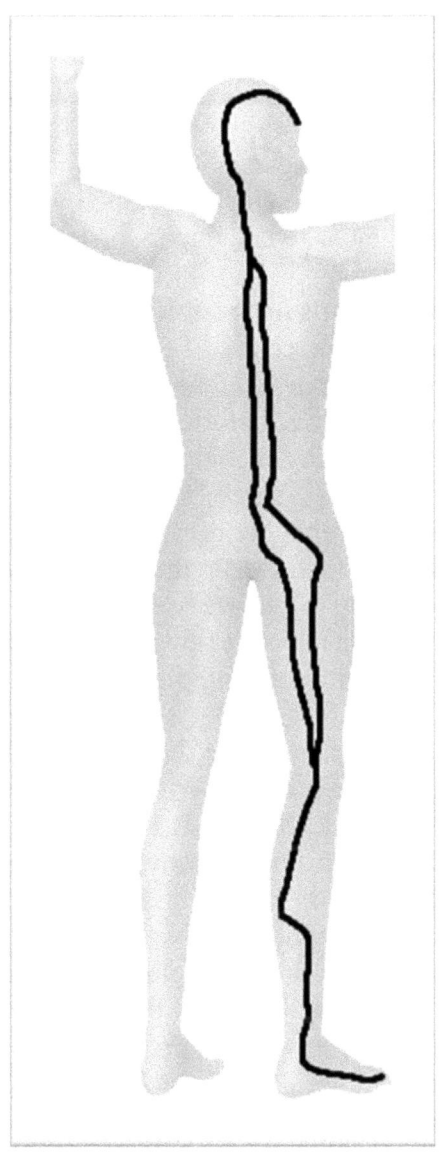

Fig. 16 The Bladder Channel.

Kidney Qi is associated with our bones and nervous system and also provides our 'get up and go' energy, basic vitality and creativity. Kidney Qi also governs our ears and sense of hearing. It is paired with the Bladder Channel and so is also involved in controlling excretion. The location of the Bladder Channel and Kidney Qi's association with bones and nerves mean that they are very important for avoiding back problems.

The Kidney Channel starts on the sole of the foot at the 'Bubbling Spring' point in the centre of the ball of the foot (this is the only acupoint on the sole of the foot). It then flows up across the instep of the foot before passing behind the medial malleolus (again the bony sticking out bit on the inside of the ankle!) where it makes a small 'loop' before flowing up the inside of the leg (towards the back of the leg). From the groin, the Kidney Channel flows up the front of the body a short distance to the side of the centre line. It moves a little further away from the centre line as it flows up the chest (but still towards the centre line from the nipple) and finishes just below the clavicle.

The Bladder Channel starts beside the corner of the eye (closest to the centre line) and flows over the top of the head and down the back of the neck a little to the side of the centre line. It then continues to flow downwards along two pathways alongside the spine (one closer and one further from the spine). These two flows continue down the centre of the back of the leg and reconvene into a single flow at the back of the knee before continuing down to the middle of the gastrocnemius muscle in the lower leg. From the base of the gastrocnemius (the large muscle at the back of your calf) it moves onto the outside of the leg (still towards the back 'edge' of the leg) and passes behind the lateral malleolus (the bony bit on the outside of the ankle). It then flows along the little toe edge of the foot before finishes next to the toenail on the little toe. The Bladder Channel is the longest of the twelve Channels.

Qigong exercises for Kidney Qi usually involve leaning forwards or backwards to stretch the front or back of the body or involve leg stretches that stretch the hamstrings. Sometimes a twisting motion of the body can be used to stretch these Channels as well.

The Tree or Wood Channels.

Liver and Gall Bladder.

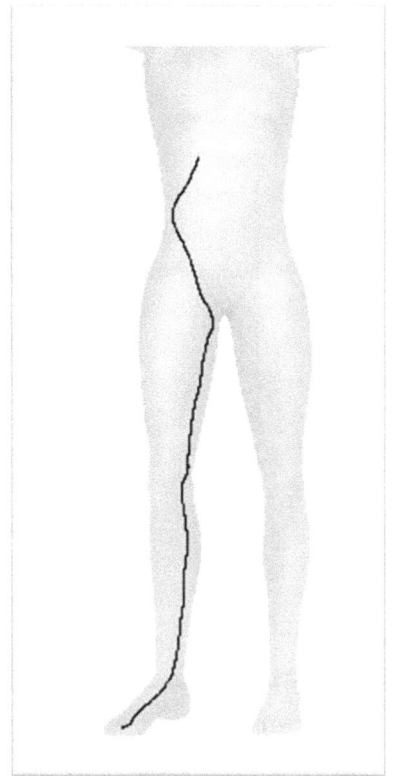

Fig. 17 The Liver Channel.

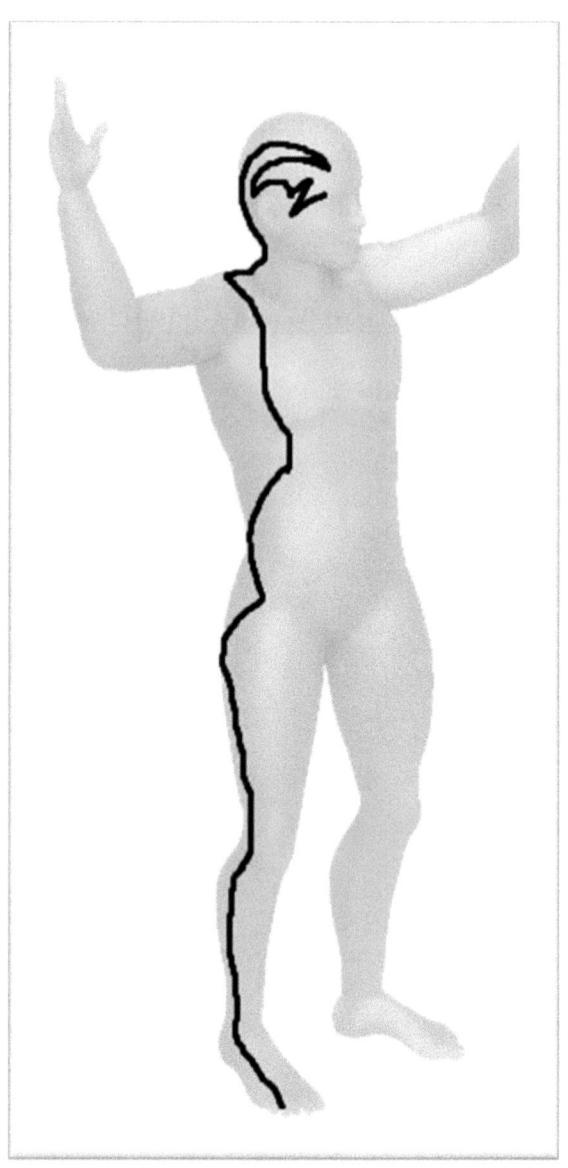

Fig. 18 The Gall Bladder Channel.

Liver Qi is associated with our ability to plan ahead, it tends to have a strong upward feel and helps us to move forwards. It is associated with flexibility, both mentally and physically as demonstrated by its role in controlling our tendons. The emotion associated with Liver Qi is anger which is often caused by frustration when things do not go according to plan. The eyes and our eyesight are governed by Liver Qi and again it is interesting to note the links with Western Medicine where it is recognized that a yellow colour in the eyes is associated with liver problems.

The Liver Channel starts beside the base of the nail of the big toe (on the side closer to the little toe), it then flows along the big toe side of the top of the foot towards the outside of the ankle. It flows in front of the medial malleolus and then continues up the inside of the leg (it is easiest to think of it as just passing up the middle of the inside of the leg between the Spleen and Kidney Channels). From the groin, it flows up and to the side of the body above the hip before heading back towards the centre line to finish at the edge of the ribcage below and slightly towards the side of the body from the nipple.

The Gall Bladder Channel begins close to the corner of the eye (on the side towards the ear), it then flows towards the ear before passing above and around to the base of the skull behind the ear. It then curves back up and onto the forehead before heading back again towards the back of the neck (so it follows a 'zigzagging' path across the side of the head). It flows down to the rear of the side of the neck and then onto the top of the shoulder before passing down to the side of the body (flowing in front of the arm). The Gall Bladder Channel then 'zigzags' again as it passes down the side of the body until it reaches the side of the buttock (where you can feel a dip in the muscle). It then flows down the middle of the outside of the leg before passing just in front of the lateral malleolus and then along the top of the little toe edge of the foot (so above the Bladder Channel). It finishes beside the base of the nail of the toe next to the little toe (on the side closest to the little toe).

Qigong exercises that benefit Tree Qi involve leaning to the sides and twisting movements so they are often also linked to Earth Qi exercises. Many Qigong exercises are therefore described as being beneficial for both Spleen and Liver. Some Liver Qigong exercises are characterized by actively 'glaring' with the eyes as a way of accentuating the Liver Qi rather than the Spleen Qi within the exercise.

Channel locations for Qigong Practice.

For practical purposes, whilst doing Qigong, it is not necessary to remember the exact path each Channel takes through the body. It is, however, useful to remember where on the hands and feet each Channel starts or ends and the general aspect of the torso and each limb through which each Channel flows. Note that the following images use the 'short-hand' initials to identify each Channel (HT – Heart, SI – Small Intestine, HP – Heart Protector, TH – Triple Heater, SP – Spleen, ST – Stomach, LG – Lung, LI – Large Intestine, KD – Kidney, BL – Bladder, LV – Liver and GB – Gall Bladder).

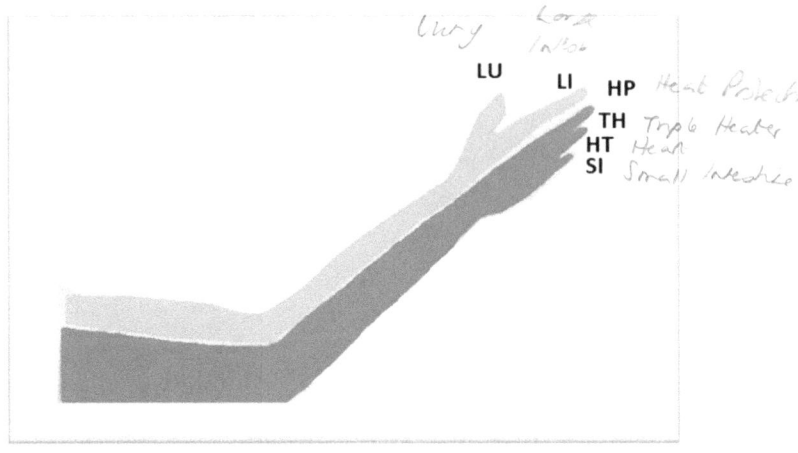

Fig. 19 The Channels of the arm.

As we can see from figure nineteen above, the Fire Channels flow along the middle and little finger edge of the arms and the Metal Channels flow along the thumb edge. This is the same for both the underside and outer side of the arm.

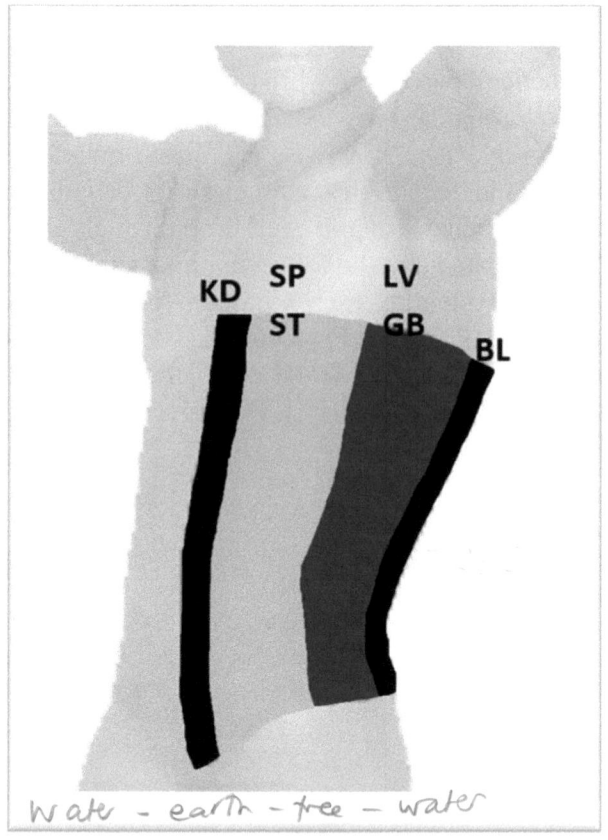

Fig. 20 The Channels on the torso.

On the torso, the Tree Channels flow more on the sides of the body. The Earth Channels are also located to the sides but can be considered to come more onto the front of the body. The Water Channels are generally considered to be more associated with the back of the body (chiefly due to the Bladder Channel flowing down either side of the spine and covering much of the back) but note that the Kidney Channel does run up the front of the body near to the centre line.

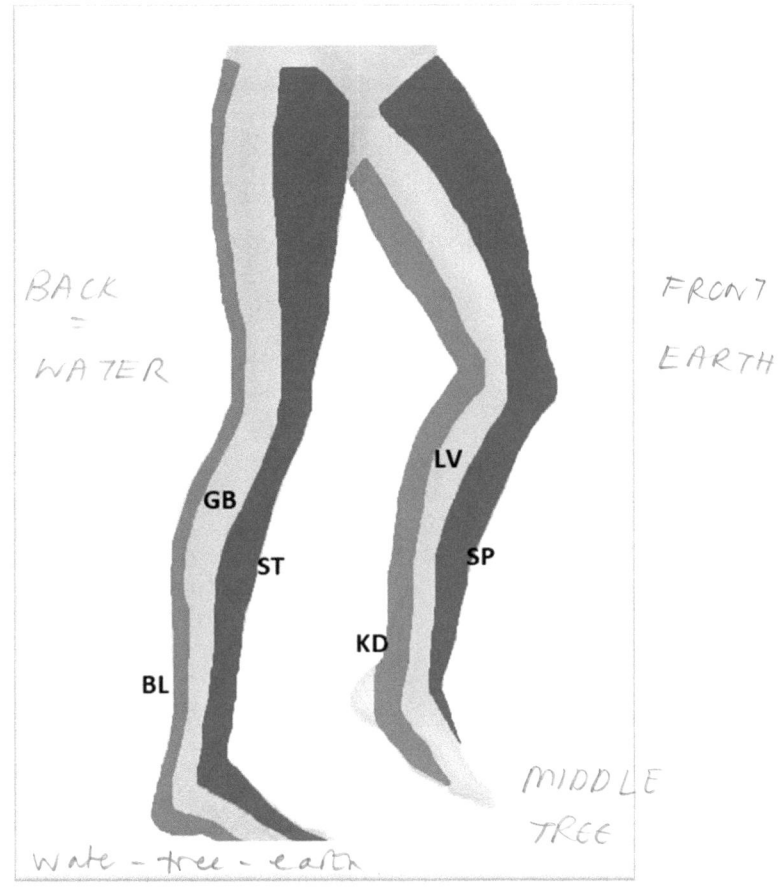

Fig. 21 The Channels of the legs.

When it comes to the legs, you can consider the back of the legs to relate to the Water Channels, the front of the legs relates more to the Earth Channels and the Tree Channels flow along the middle of the outside and inside of each leg.

Chapter Six.

The 'Extraordinary Vessels'.

Reservoirs of Qi

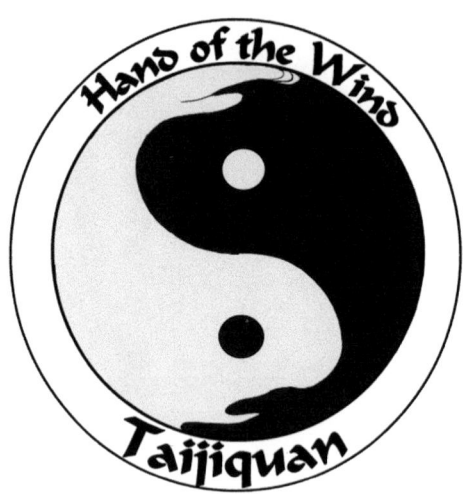

Conception
Govenor
Thrusting
Girdle
Heel (x2)
Linking (x2)

As well as the twelve Channels which are associated with particular organ functions and the Five Transformations there are eight other 'Vessels' recognized as of importance in Chinese Medicine and therefore in Qigong practice. These 'Vessels' primarily serve as reservoirs for Qi which can then be distributed through the body via the Channels. Unlike the Twelve Channels they do not always flow in a particular direction (and sometimes within Qigong practice we aim to determine the directions in which they flow) and most of them do not have acupoints along their lengths. The lack of acupoints specifically linked to the 'Extraordinary Vessels' (sometimes referred to as 'Special Vessels') means that they are less well known in the West where Acupuncture is the main driving force for knowledge of how Qi flows in the body.

The two Vessels that do have their own acupoints are the most well-known in the West and they are the Conception and Governor Vessels. The other six are the Girdle Vessel, the Thrusting Vessel, the two Heel Vessels and the two Linking Vessels. They all have important functions within the body and should all be considered when practicing Qigong in order to achieve maximum benefits.

The Conception Vessel.

The Conception Vessel (CV, 'Ren Mai') 'begins' at the centre of the perineum (halfway between the genitals and the anus), although do remember the Qi could flow either way within it. The Vessel then runs up the centre line of the front of the body to finish at the centre of the 'groove' beneath the mouth (it does then split around the mouth and continue up the cheeks to the eyes, but this is less important for our purposes).

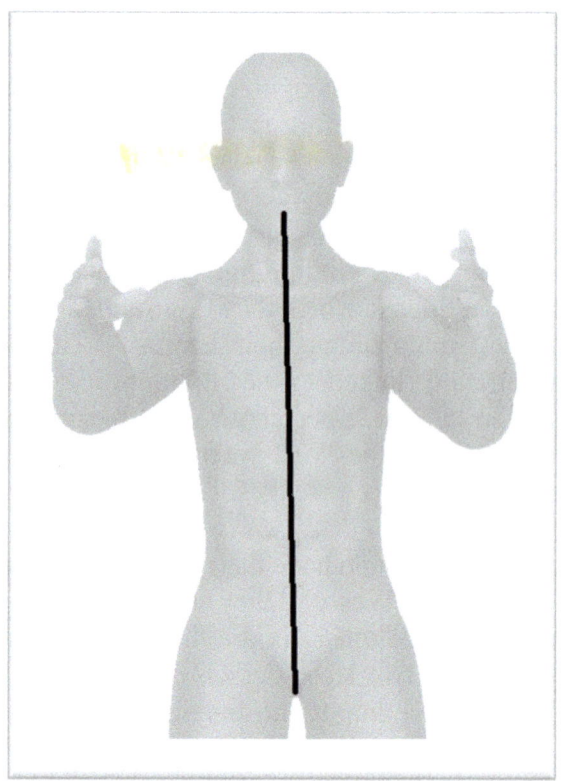

Fig. 22 The Conception Vessel.

The Conception Vessel serves as the main 'reservoir' of Qi for distribution among the Yin Channels and therefore plays a role in controlling the Qi in those Channels. It is also involved in sexual and reproductive health and is often used in acupuncture to treat fertility issues.

The Governor Vessel.

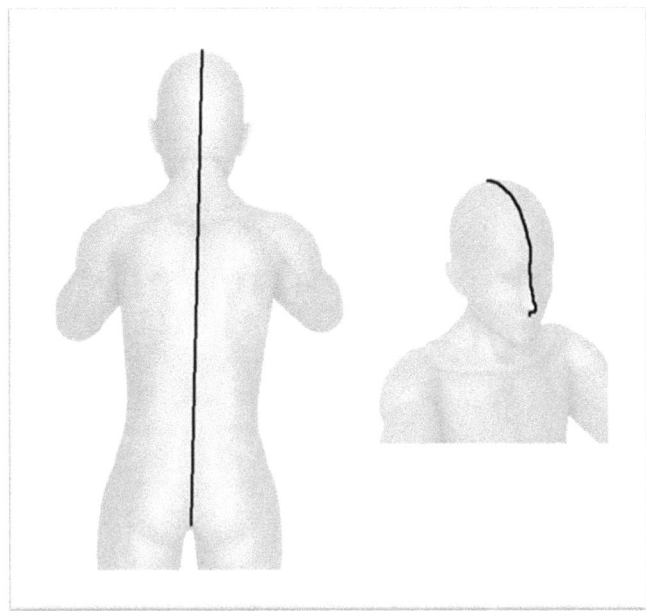

Fig. 23 The Governor Vessel.

Governor Vessel (GV or 'Du Mai') 'begins' just behind the anus and runs up the centre line of the back of the body. It continues over the top of the head and then down along the nose to the mouth, finishing inside the mouth just above the front teeth.

Just as the Conception Vessel serves to distribute Qi amongst the Yin Channels, the Governor Vessel serves the same purpose for the Yang Channels of the body. As the Governor Vessel runs along the line of the spine, it is not surprising that it is involved with maintaining the health of the spine and is therefore often used in acupuncture to treat back problems.

The Thrusting Vessel.

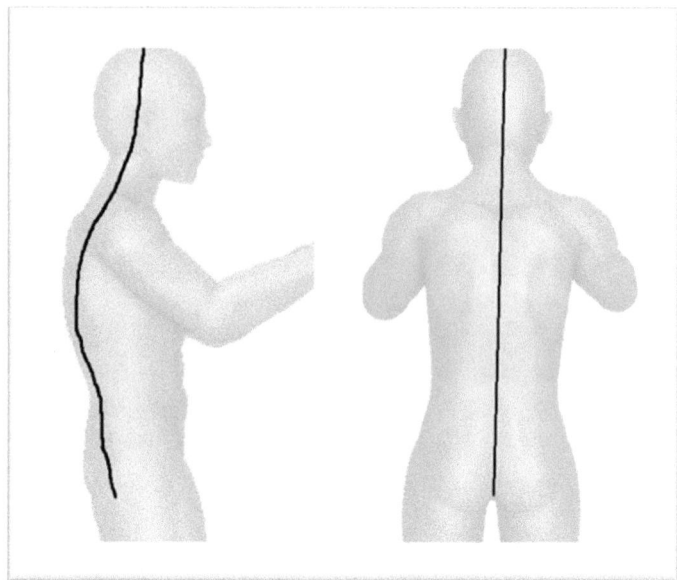

Fig. 24 The Thrusting Vessel.

The Thrusting Vessel runs directly along the spinal cord (within the spine) from the top of the head directly down to the perineum. For practical purposes, some Qigong teachings describe it as flowing up through the centre of the body (which would place it in front of the spine). As with the other 'Extraordinary Vessels', it serves as a reservoir for Qi and helps to distribute Qi within the body. The Thrusting Vessel connects directly to the Kidney Channels and is therefore very important in helping to maintain our vitality and core energy levels. Within Qigong training, the Thrusting Vessel is used in techniques involved in 'nourishing the Marrow' and helps to maintain the upward feeling of 'buoyancy' that sustains our posture.

The Girdle Vessel.

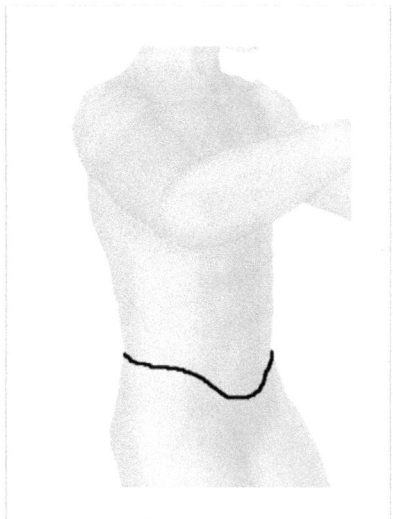

Fig. 25 The Girdle Vessel.

The Girdle or Belt Vessel encircles the body horizontally (uniquely amongst all the Channels or Vessels!), it runs just below the ribs at the sides of the body, across the lower back and then lower across the front of the abdomen.

The Girdle Vessel helps to regulate Qi across the different 'halves' of the body – both vertically and horizontally. It can distribute energy from one side of the body to the other and is also involved with the flow of Qi upwards and downwards through the body. Weakness in the Girdle Vessel can lead to lower back pain and can have an impact on balance (physically, mentally and emotionally!). Within Tai Chi training, with its emphasis on 'waist', the Girdle Vessel is constantly being strengthened and exercised.

The Heel Vessels.

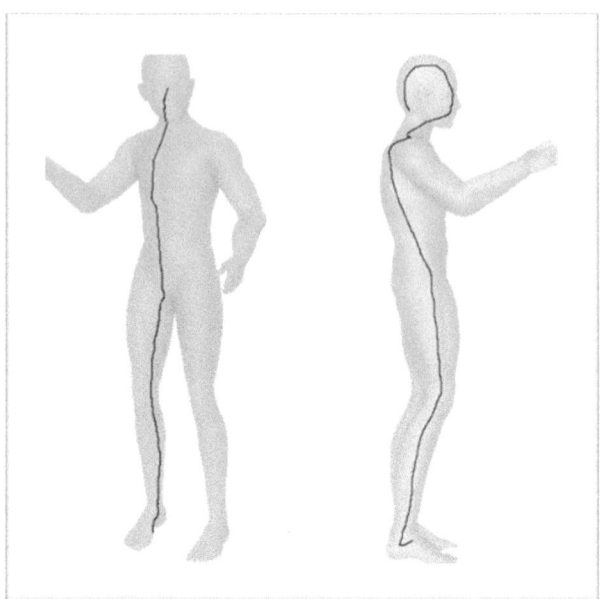

Fig. 26 The Yin and Yang Heel Vessels.

The Yin and Yang Heel Vessels form a 'circuit' within each side of the body and are considered to be important in regulating the balance of Qi between the Yin and Yang Channels. The location of the Yin Heel Vessel is along the inside of the leg and up through the body to the shoulder and then to the eye (following the course of the Kidney Channel for much of this distance). The Yang Heel Vessel flows down the side of the body and the outside of the leg (from the base of the skull to the eye and then to the heel). These Vessels are involved in both our 'grounding' and our ability to move our feet and therefore are very important to be considered in all the 'stance-work' that we use within our Tai Chi and Qigong practice.

The Linking Vessels.

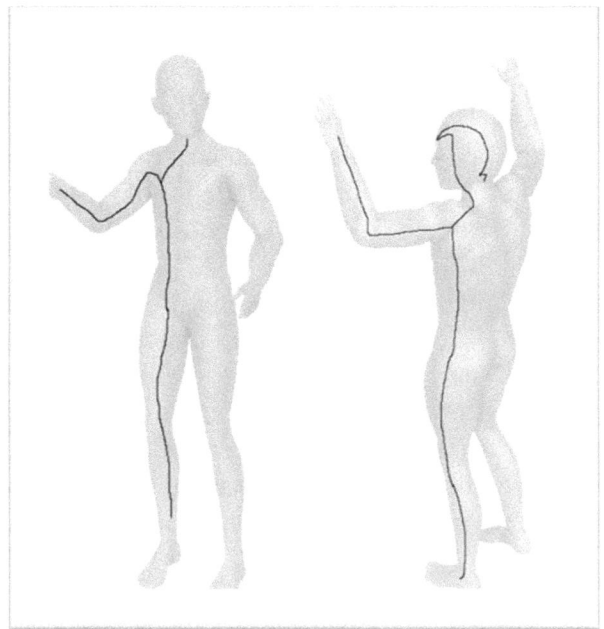

Fig. 27 The Yin and Yang Linking Vessels.

As with the Heel Vessels, there are both Yin and Yang Linking Vessels and each are found on both sides of the body. The Yin Linking Vessel connects the Yin Channels of the body, starting from the inner side of the lower leg, it runs up the inner front aspect of the thigh and then up the side of the abdomen to the chest where it traverses inwards to meet the Conception Vessel.

The Yang Linking Vessel runs from the Governor Vessel at the base of the skull onto the side of the head. It flows up the top of the side of the head to the forehead and then back down the side of the head behind the ear to the neck. From the side of the neck, it flows outwards onto the shoulder before flowing down the side of the body and leg to finish below the back of the ankle on the outside of the heel.

Both the Yin and Yang Linking Vessels also connect to the Channels of the arms, with the Yang Linking Vessel connecting to the Triple Heater Channel and the Yin with the Heart Protector. The Yang Linking Vessels connect the Yang Channels of the body, and along with the Yin Linking Vessels are responsible for maintaining the balance of Qi between the Yin and Yang Channels.

There are many specific Qigong training techniques which utilize and enhance the functioning of the Extraordinary Vessels but most of these techniques are beyond the remit of this book and should only be practiced under the supervision of an experienced and qualified teacher. One technique which is integral to our Tai Chi training is the 'Microcosmic Orbit' which we shall look at in the next chapter.

Chapter Seven.

The 'Microcosmic Orbit'.

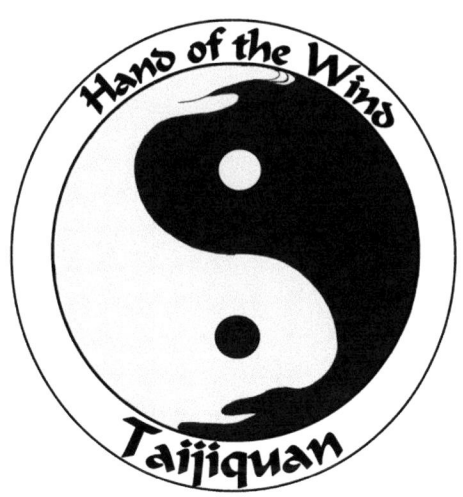

Normally, as adults the Qi within the Conception Vessel, the Governor Vessel and the Thrusting Vessel tends to flow in a particular way as shown in the following diagram.

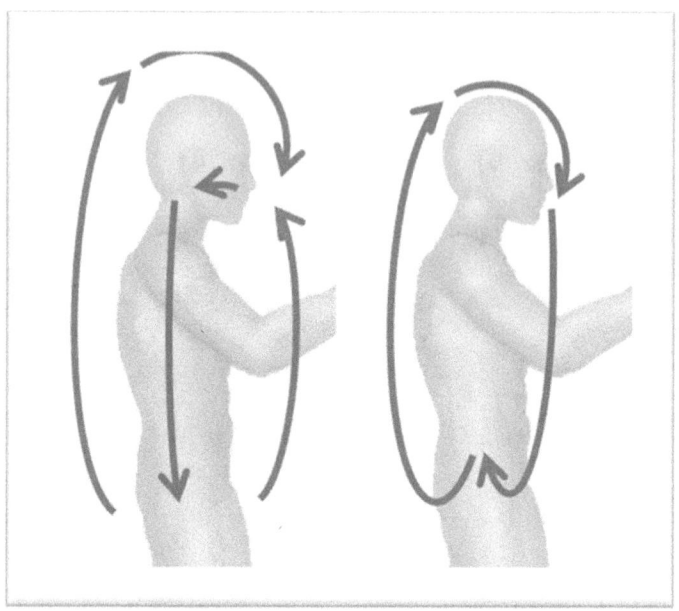

Fig. 28 'Normal' adult flow of Qi through CV, GV and Thrusting Vessel (on left) and the 'Microcosmic Orbit' (on the right).

However, when we were young children, the Qi flowed differently by forming a circuit between the Conception and Governor Vessels, flowing down the Conception Vessel on the front of the body and then up the Governor Vessel on the back of the body. We call this circulation the 'Microcosmic Orbit' and within our Tai Chi and Qigong training we aim to revert the flow to this earlier state. In simple terms, this can be considered as a means of 'rejuvenating' our Qi and helping our bodies to 'remember' the vitality and healing ability they had when we were very young. An aspect of the Microcosmic Orbit which is often not taught is that the Qi flows up from the end of the Conception Vessel into the Tantien and then back down to the start of the Governor Vessel as shown in figure twenty-eight.

There is one very important thing to consider, in order for the Microcosmic Orbit to form – it is vital that the tip of the tongue is in contact with the top of the mouth. This is something that you will need to be aware of initially but becomes habitual and subconscious with practice. The tip of the tongue curls upwards to contact the top of the mouth, as if about to pronounce the sound of the letter 'L'. On a martial note, it also ensures that your tongue does not get caught between your teeth and bitten!

The Microcosmic Orbit also has the effect of 'freeing' the Thrusting Vessel so that it can adopt the upward flow which helps to nourish our brains and maintain our posture with the feeling of 'buoyancy' that we talk about within the Tai Chi Form. It is very important to note that if we adopt an upward flow of Qi within the Thrusting Vessel, we must ensure an equivalent downward flow to prevent Qi stagnating in our heads. This can be achieved by circulating the Qi from the Thrusting Vessel back into the Microcosmic Orbit and by utilizing the Yang Heel and Linking Vessels to draw the Qi back downwards.

In order to activate the Microcosmic Orbit, we regularly use meditation (usually standing or seated) and guide the Qi into the circulation with our minds by using visualization techniques. It is also interesting to note that the first sequence of the Lee Family Tai Chi Form is designed to activate the Microcosmic Orbit which should then be maintained throughout our practice of the Tai Chi Form.

Chapter Eight.

The 'Gates'.

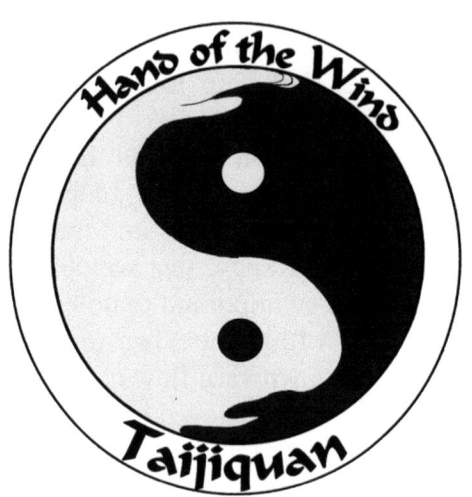

Along the twelve Channels (and also the Conception Vessel and Governor Vessel), there are many points which can be used to access and manipulate the flow of Qi within the body and this forms the basis of acupuncture and acupressure. For the purposes of Tai Chi and Qigong training, it is not necessary to know the locations and uses of all of these acupoints but there are a few points that we do regularly utilize in our training.

These points are particularly useful for allowing Qi to flow into and out of the body and we therefore refer to them as the 'Gates'. You should aim to learn the locations of these Gates and be aware of how they align with each other when you practice Tai Chi or Qigong exercises. Practice standing meditation and focus on these points in order to learn their locations, be aware of how they align in different Standing Qigong postures and build your awareness of how they can nourish each other.

Initially, practice Standing Qigong with the palms of the hands facing each other (Lao Gong point directed towards the Lao Gong point of the other hand), also experiment with lining up Lao Gong with Qi Hu or He Gu with Qi Hu and try adjusting the distance between the points as you breathe. Expand the distance as you breathe in and contract the distance as you breathe out. Over time, consider each Qigong exercise and each posture within the Tai Chi Form to explore the Gates and how they interact with each other.

The table on the next page gives the names and locations for each of the Gates and is followed by illustrations to assist with their locations.

Gate	Location	Channel
Bubbling Spring (Yong Quan)	On the bottom of the ball of the foot.	Kidney (KD 1)
Lao Gong	In the centre of the palm of the hand.	Heart Protector (HP 8)
He Gu	On the bulge of muscle between the base of the thumb and the forefinger.	Large Intestine (LI 4)
Qi Hu	On the front of the body, just below the centre of the clavicle.	Stomach (ST 13)
Yang Gu	The little finger edge of the wrist.	Small Intestine (SI 5)
Huan Tiao	On the side of the buttock, where the gluteus maximus muscle meets the hip joint.	Gall Bladder (GB 30)
Lower Tantien	On the centre line of the front of the body, 2 inches below the navel.	Conception Vessel (CV 4)
Middle Tantien	On the centre line of the front of the body, in the mid-point of the sternum.	Conception Vessel (CV 17)
Upper Tantien	On the centre line of the front of the forehead, the 'third eye' point.	Governor Vessel (Not a numbered point)
Bai Hui	On the top of the head, on the centre line.	Governor Vessel (GV 20)
Hui Yin	On the centre line, half-way between the genitals and anus.	Conception Vessel (CV 1)
Ming Men	Between the 2nd and 3rd Lumbar vertebrae in the lower back.	GV4

64

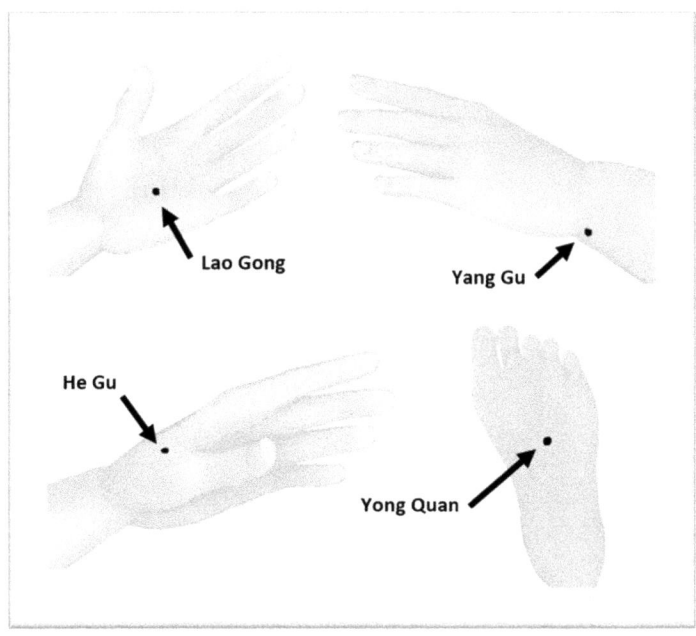

Fig. 29 The 'Gates' located on the hands and feet.

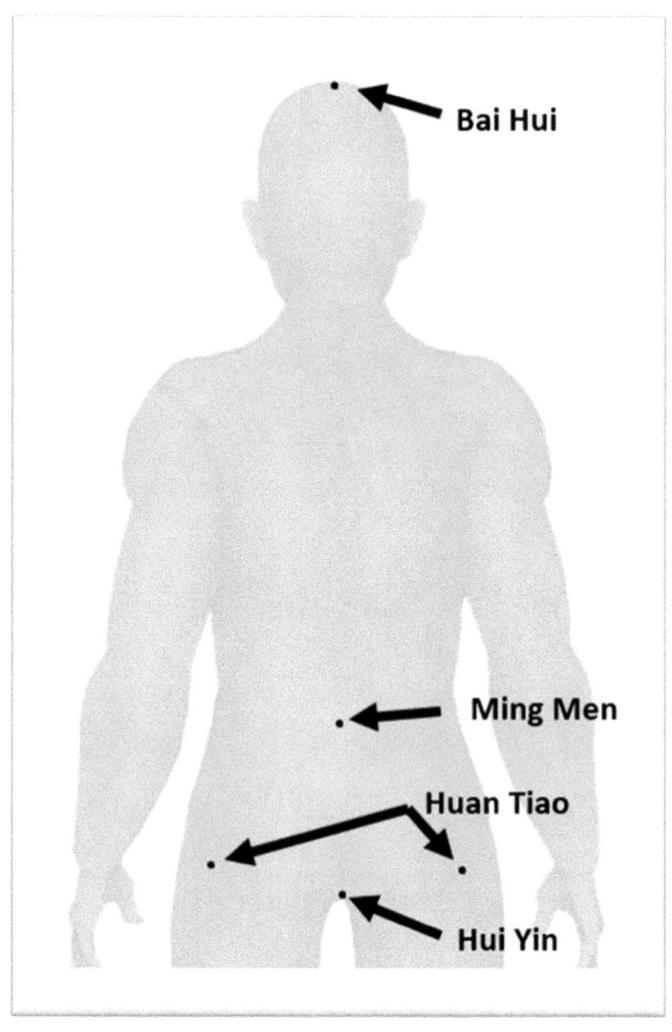

Fig. 30 The 'Gates' of the back of the body.

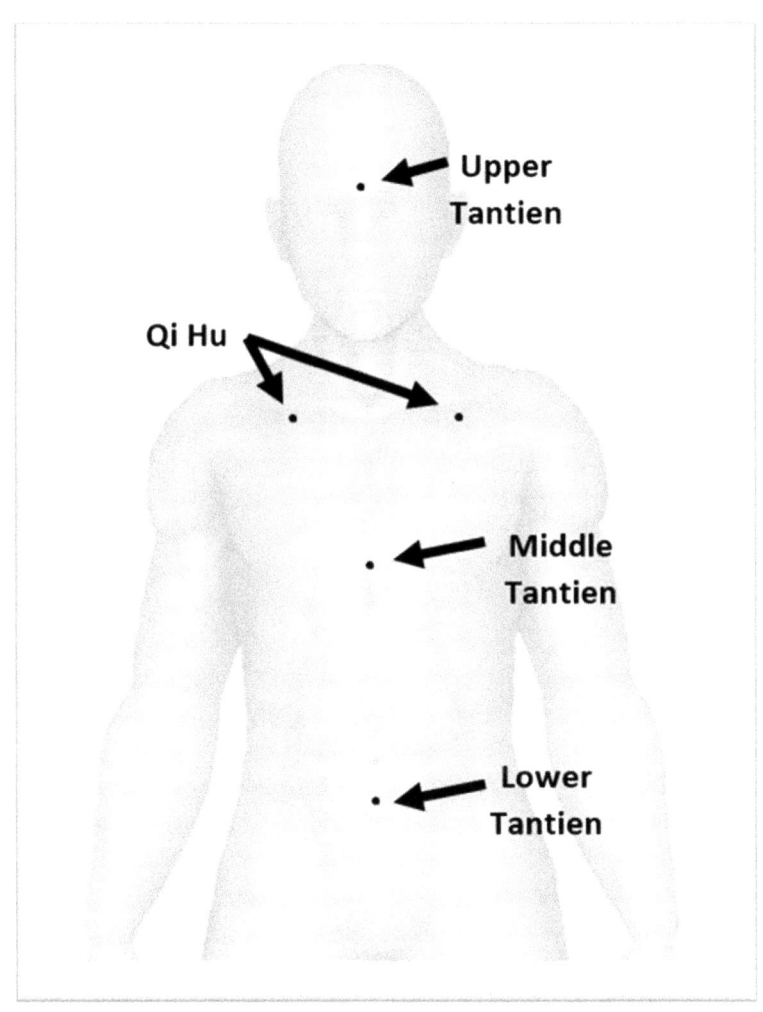

Fig. 31 The 'Gates' of the front of the body.

Chapter Nine.

Posture and Limbs.

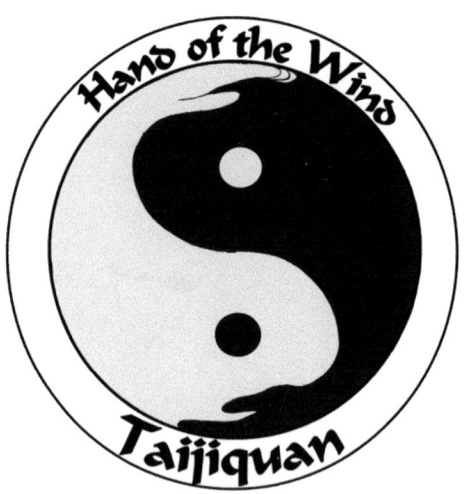

Posture.

Remember that we use the term 'posture' to refer to the position and alignment of the body from the waist upwards and the specific posture we adopt depends upon the exercise that we are practicing. However, there are a few basic points to always bear in mind to ensure that we use a correct posture.

Firstly, the tailbone (coccyx) should be 'tucked' underneath the body bringing the pelvis into a better alignment with the spine. This takes the pressure off the lower back by opening and straightening the joints between the pelvis and the spine (the sacroiliac joint and also the joints between the sacrum and the lumber spine as well as the joints between the vertebrae of the lumber spine itself). By adjusting the alignment of the coccyx, we provide a good foundation for the spine to rest upon and therefore adopt its correct (gently curved) alignment. Standing with the knees locked or hyperextended and wearing high-heeled shoes are both particularly detrimental to the correct alignment of the pelvis.

It is also common for the chest to be sunken downwards, pulling the head forwards and exaggerating the curve in the thoracic spine and this is also something we should be aware of and avoid. Usually students of Tai Chi and Qigong are advised to hold the head as if it is suspended from the highest point of the crown to encourage a good alignment of the upper spine. As the head is held upwards (requiring a good flow of Qi through the Thrusting Vessel), the chin is allowed to drop slightly which opens up the cervical spine (the bones of the neck). The following illustrations contrast an incorrect posture with the correct posture we are aiming for in our Tai Chi and Qigong practice (and therefore in the rest of our lives as well!).

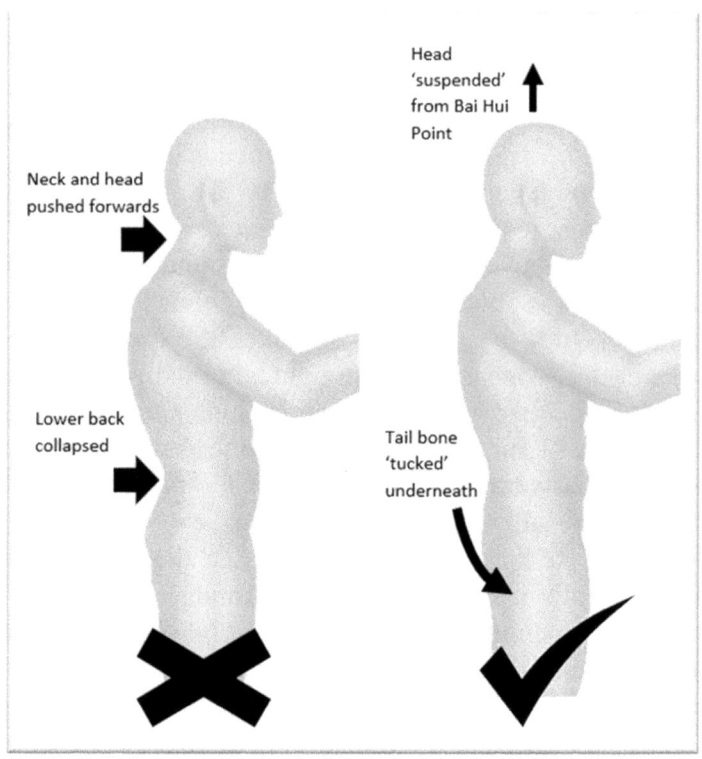

Fig. 32 Incorrect and correct posture of the spine.

The Limbs.

Once we adopt a correct posture by aligning the pelvis and spine, we need to consider our limbs. The key thing to remember is that we should never fully lock the elbow or knee joints by fully straightening (or by hyperextending) the arm or leg. When the joints are locked, Qi flow is restricted and unnecessary tension is introduced into the body. And from a martial perspective, a locked limb will quickly become a broken limb! It is also important to not over-flex a joint and it is often said that elbows should never adopt a tighter angle than ninety degrees. Also be aware that the wrists should not be too bent in any direction – as a guide you should not usually see deep 'creases' appear in the skin at the wrists. Wrists, elbows and knees are relatively easy to be aware of and monitor for tension in these ways but also be aware of how you are using your ankles, hips and shoulders.

With regards to hips and shoulders, be particularly aware when raising the arms or legs to ensure that the joint is not adversely affected. When raising a leg into Crane, Dog or Horse stances for example it is important the thigh is not raised too high (parallel to the floor is definitely too high!). When the arms are raised, the shoulders should not 'lift' – be aware of the interaction between the thoracic spine in the upper back and the shoulder to monitor for tension in the shoulders. Often when the arms raise up in front of the body to head height or higher, the arms really only raise to shoulder height and then the chest 'opens' upwards to bring the hands higher as shown in the following illustrations.

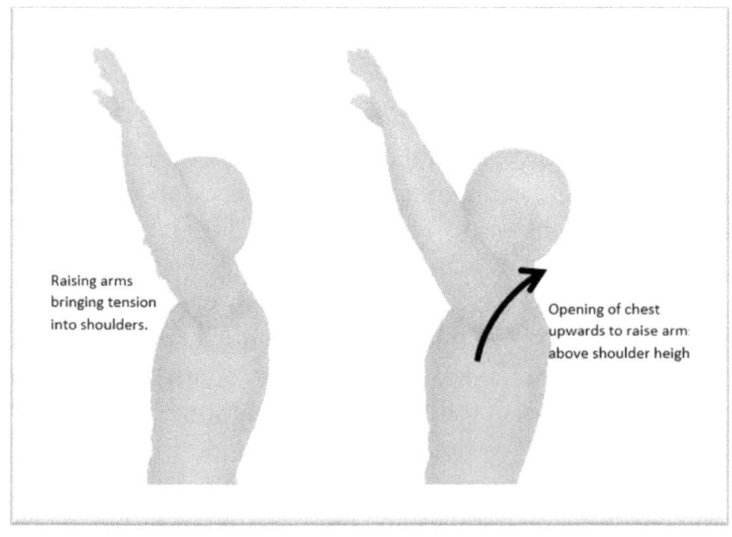

Fig. 33 Lifting the arms above shoulder height.

To get the idea of this 'opening' of the chest upwards, first bring your arms up in front of your body to chest height with the palms facing away from the body and the fingertips towards each other (as in move number two of the Lee Family Tai Chi Form). Then, continue to bring your arms upwards to higher than shoulder height – be aware of the levels of tension in the shoulders. Now, bring the arms up to shoulder height again in the same way and this time think about lifting up through the front of the body so that the chest lifts and 'opens' upwards. Allow the head to move with the upper back and neck so that you naturally look upwards but be careful not to collapse and compress any part of the back – the entire lifting feeling should come from the spine opening upwards and not from leaning backwards. This is both supported by and encourages the upward flow of Qi within the Thrusting Vessel that we refer to as 'buoyancy'.

72

Be aware that correct spinal posture and pelvis alignment are connected to the correct use of the limbs. For example, when the pelvis is properly aligned in Dragon Stance it becomes impossible for the rear leg to be fully straightened. When the spine is correctly aligned upon the good foundation of a correctly aligned pelvis, then the shoulders can relax and allow the arms to 'hang' from the central support of the spine.

Chapter Ten.

Stances and Stepping.

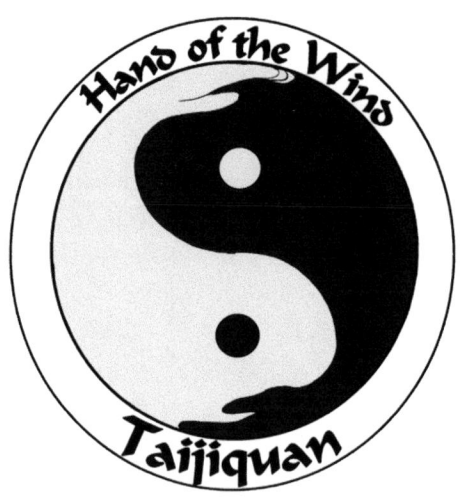

We use the term 'stance' to describe the alignment of the body from the waist downwards including foot position, weight distribution and the interaction and alignment of the joints of the lower limbs. This book is not intended to teach the various stances that we use within our Tai Chi and Qigong training and does not contain descriptions of the stances (they are described in other Hand of the Wind publications). This book is intended to encourage students of Tai Chi and Qigong to think deeper about their stances and therefore this section will focus on the common aspects that should be considered in all stances.

Firstly, as explained in the previous chapter, it is essential that the knees are never 'locked'. Examine the alignment of the joints within each of your stances carefully to ensure that they are never over-extended or flexed too far. This includes being aware of the angles of the feet within Eagle and Leopard stances for example and the angle of the rear foot in Dragon, Snake and Duck stances. Consider how the angle of the ankle joint affects the muscles of the entire leg and therefore the flow of Qi through the Channels within each leg.

The weight should be slightly forward onto the balls of the feet – but not too much! So, when standing, the weight of the body should not press down through the mid-point of the foot (length-wise), but should be more towards the toes so that you feel the grounding through the ball of the foot and the Bubbling Spring point. Do not over-extend the weight too far forwards however – the heel should still be securely on the floor. You should feel 'grounded' but also should feel that you have some 'bounce' in your feet and an ability to move freely.

When it comes to moving the feet, there are two main 'rules' that we need to follow: never move a weighted foot and always step heel-toe. It seems like an obvious statement to say that you need to move the weight out of a foot before you can step that foot into a new position, but it is often the case that many students do not fully free up the foot before stepping and therefore introduce extra tension into the body as they step. It is common for beginners to shift the weight out of a foot by simple shifting their pelvis to the side but this is a linear movement and again introduces unwanted tension. Consider how the centre (focusing on the Lower Tantien) moves in a subtle (do not exaggerate it!) circle to allow the weight to shift in a more relaxed fashion. This will lead to the more relaxed 'circular' stepping style that you will find in many martial arts, but again care must be taken to ensure that this is not exaggerated.

Students adopting a more circular approach to weight shifts during stepping will also tend to begin to appreciate the importance of relaxing through the groin or inguinal area. Along with the relaxed opening and closing of the chest, the relaxation and movement through this inguinal area is a key element of the integration of Yin and Yang within our Tai Chi and Qigong. It is therefore very important that students do not become rigid within their stances and that they allow the subtle movements in the hip joints that are needed to utilize the stances correctly and to be able to step in a relaxed manner.

Once the weight is shifted to allow the foot to move, it is important to place the foot correctly onto the ground – this should always be controlled without any sense of 'falling' into the foot. Within Lee Style Tai Chi and Qigong training, the foot should always be placed onto the ground heel first and then the foot allowed to settle onto the floor with the ball of the foot and then the toes lying onto the ground. Some texts refer to the feeling of 'gripping' the floor with the toes but this often tends to lead to students tightening up and tensing the toes. Think of this more as the toes 'settling' onto the floor and then relaxing the pads of the toes back towards the foot and you will get the sense of a relaxed 'gripping' feeling.

The foot should still have the feeling of stepping 'heel-toe' even if the heel or ball of foot never come into contact with the ground (for example in one-legged stances such as Crane or Dog, or in stances like Cat or Monkey). The feeling within the muscles of the leg should be the same as when the foot is placed onto the floor.

Often students find it difficult to step backwards 'heel-toe' and this is likely to be caused by one of two things. Firstly, ensure that you are not 'over-stepping' – if the step is too big or long then it becomes difficult to align the joints properly to allow the heel-toe step. Otherwise, it may be that the weight has not been shifted out of the stepping foot correctly and that may require some consideration.

You should practice standing in each of your stances for reasonable periods of time (suitable to your own health and fitness) so that you can feel where the tensions arise. You can then make adjustments to find the most relaxed position within the context of each stance. As you train over the years and your body changes, your stances will also change – so this needs to be a continual process throughout all of the years of your training.

As you become comfortable in your stances you should then practice stepping in each stance. Firstly, focus on stepping and staying in the same stance (for example 'box' steps in Bear stance or 'ladder' steps in Snake stance) making sure you can comfortably step forwards, backwards, to each side and turn through a variety of angles both 'clockwise' and 'anti-clockwise'. When stepping, remember to step the front foot first when moving forwards or the back foot first when stepping backwards (unless in a neutral stance such as Bear where you should ensure you practice stepping each foot first). When stepping sideways or turning you should step the appropriate foot first (so if going left, the left foot steps first etc.).

Once you can comfortably step whilst maintaining a single stance, you should practice stepping between stances so from Bear to Dragon for example. Practice stepping between all the different stances until you feel comfortable stepping from any stance into any other stance at any angle. This is why I often tell my students that stepping practice is one of the best things that they can do – it is a huge area to study with infinite variations and many things that need to be perfected! For health training purposes, it is generally only necessary to train 'single steps' where we step the feet one at a time – 'double steps' where both feet move at the same time (jumping!) is more useful for the martial student as it develops explosive power.

Chapter Eleven.

The 'Double Weighted' Conundrum.

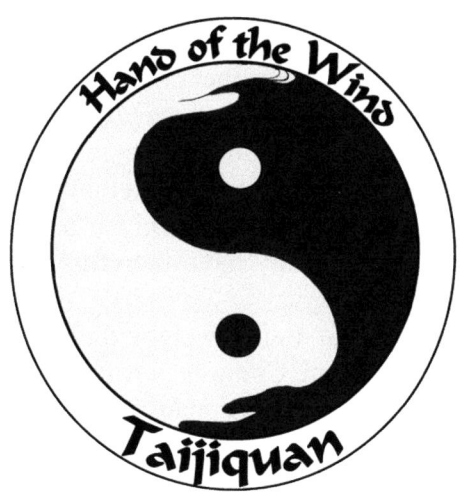

The term 'double-weighted' is often used within the context of Tai Chi and can often cause considerable amounts of confusion. In recent years, many practitioners of Tai Chi have taken the view that 'double-weighted' means having the weight of the body supported equally on both feet and this can cause issues for students of our Lee Family System where so called double-weighted stances such as Riding Horse or Snake stance are commonly employed within the Forms.

This very literal interpretation of the term 'double-weighted' seems to have its origins in the teachings of Yang Chengfu in the first half of the Twentieth Century, where he taught that the Riding Horse stance was incorrect and should not be used because it is 'double-weighted'. It is of interest to note that this may have been an attempt by the Yang family to hide the 'secrets' of their Tai Chi Ch'uan from their more public teachings and may have therefore been a deliberate misinformation strategy.

To consider what double weighted really means, as usual when translating from Chinese, we need to be aware that often a single word can carry many meanings. So, weighted could also mean emphasis rather than the physical force of gravity working on mass. This means that we need to be thinking deeper than just the superficial, physical level when we consider our Tai Chi. Double weighted could therefore be thought of as double emphasized and this can then be more easily applied to all aspects of our Tai Chi, rather than just the physical.

To return to the physical as an example, if we consider the concept of double emphasized, we then come to the idea that being in a Riding Horse stance is not incorrect but extending our weight too far forwards in a Dragon stance would be incorrect. Chee Soo used to explain double weighted as having the weight on one leg and then extending the arms both to that side as well. This is clearly an overemphasized situation and therefore incorrect. For the

80

purposes of training Tai Chi and Qigong for health, it is useful to be aware of not overextending oneself physically in any direction. For the martial student, the physical aspects of double weighted-ness become a much more complex and involved area of study, where your own body and forces must be considered in light of their interactions with your opponent(s) as well. This forms much of the in-depth study of Push Hands or Sticky Hands training for the martial student.

When considering double weighted-ness, it is essential that you also consider the concepts of Yin and Yang. Many teachers of Tai Chi will often use the concept of 'full' and 'empty' when talking about the weight distribution through the legs, but again this far too often becomes purely about weight. If we think about how the concept of Yin and Yang relates to weight distribution then the idea of full and empty becomes inadequate to describe what is really going on.

If I shift my weight into a Dragon stance from a Snake stance then more weight will be pressed down through the front foot and less weight will press down into the rear foot. But which foot is therefore Yang and which is Yin? If I consider Yang to be heavy and Yin to be light then is the front foot Yang? If I think about where is the forward movement generated from, then am I pushing backwards through the rear foot which would make the rear foot Yang? If I consider what is happening at the knee, then the front knee is flexing more (Yin) and the back knee is extending (Yang). Or consider the inguinal region where the groin on the rear leg side is opening more (Yang) as the front leg side closes more (Yin). It soon becomes clear that any detailed consideration of Yin and Yang can become quite confusing!

I would suggest you consider what is happening at the joints of the legs (ankles, knees and hips) and feel how each is opening or closing throughout any weight transfer. This is probably the easiest way to start to consider how Yin and Yang are involved in weight transfer type movements.

We also then need to consider what is happening with the Qi flow through the legs and feet as we make the same movement. Again, this often seems to get caught up with the physical for many people, so if the weight is on one leg the assumption is that there is more Qi being directed through that leg. This is simply not true!

When considering the flow of Qi through the Yin and Yang Channels of the legs, they should be in balance for the sake of our health! When we choose to direct Qi with our minds (Yi) for the purposes of movement, it is often therefore more useful to consider the Extraordinary Vessels.

So, standing in a Dragon stance (for example) feel the flow of Qi through the Yin and Yang Heel Vessels within each leg– extend that circular flow so that it goes into and out of the floor instead of just circulating within your body by turning at the foot. This allows you to develop a flow, not unlike the Small Microcosmic Orbit, which incorporates the legs and the ground. Then, continue the exercise by circulating the Qi down one leg and then through the floor to return up the other leg (using both sets of Heel Vessels, this does of course go both left to right and right to left simultaneously). Add this in to your stepping practice, by focusing on the upward and downward flows as you shift your weight and step each foot. With practice you will develop an improved ability to transfer your weight and step whilst maintaining your 'grounded-ness'. This will help you to avoid becoming 'stuck' in any stance – whether the weight is equally balanced in both feet or not!

The above ideas and exercises are intended to get you to start to think more about how the weight transfers between the legs without over emphasizing or 'double-weighting' any aspect of the movements.

When training Tai Chi and Qigong for health purposes it becomes quickly apparent that the weight does often shift from one leg to the other and this is often described as 'rocking'. This is another reason why many people get confused about double weighted-ness and think that it is concerned with avoiding having the weight on both legs equally. The reason we 'rock' is not about avoiding becoming 'double weighted' and stuck – it is more to do with health than the martial. If as a martial artist I am constantly shifting my weight from one leg to another, it is very easy for an opponent to time their attack for a moment when my weight is shifting towards their attack – this would be considered as double weighted with my opponent!

As we shift the weight from one leg to the other, when practicing Tai Chi or Qigong we are effectively massaging the Bubbling Spring point (Yong Quan) in the sole of the foot (the first point of the Kidney Channel). This is important in stimulating the movement of Qi throughout the Channels of the body and invigorating our Qi. It also stimulates and helps to regulate blood flow – remember that Qi follows blood and blood follows Qi!

In summary, always remember that double weighted-ness is not just about weight – it applies to all aspects of our Tai Chi and Qigong practice. The arms must not be double-weighted, the mind must not be double-weighted and so on. If you think of the term of double weighted as meaning over-emphasized or over-extended it will be far more helpful in practical terms for your training. Some teachers use the terms double Yang or double Yin or even Yin Yin and Yang Yang and these are all just different interpretations of the concept of double weighted-ness. As in all aspects of life, going to extremes creates weakness and unsustainability.

Chapter Twelve.

Grounding.

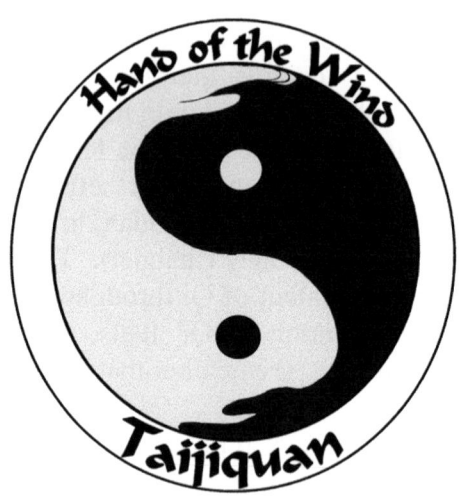

In the previous chapter, we touched upon the idea of grounded-ness which is linked to (but, importantly, not restricted to only being about) how our weight is distributed to keep us connected to the floor.

From a physical perspective, our grounded-ness is intrinsically linked to balance – our mass needs to be supported by our legs in a way that means that we are not falling over! However, much of the time people use muscular tension to counter the fact that they are not in a balanced stance. The more relaxed you are, the more grounded you will feel. As an analogy, understandable to all parents – consider the difference between picking up an awake child or a sleeping child!

This brings us back to the importance (again!) of practicing stances and stepping. Be aware of the relaxation of each muscle group within each stance and then consider the muscle changes required for stepping. Practicing the one-legged stances (Crane, Dog, Horse, Stork) and finding the correct joint alignments to maintain the optimum relaxation is necessary to understand how to move your body (and particularly your centre of mass) during stepping.

As you find the ways to relax into your stances you will enable the Qi to flow more smoothly and strongly through the legs. The exercise described in the previous chapter to circulate the Heel Vessel Qi through the ground is another important exercise for improving your grounding. Practice the same exercise in the one-legged stances, both by circulating through one leg at a time and by connecting the two legs through the ground. This will help you to understand how the foot that is not on the floor can still be involved in grounding and therefore still assists your grounding as you step a foot.

The Bubbling Spring Point on the sole of the foot is one of our 'gates' which means it is a point where it is particularly easy for Qi to pass into and out of the body. This is the point where you will naturally find yourself 'grounding' your Qi into the floor. In all stances it is vital to consider the quality of the contact between Bubbling Spring and the floor. Practice extending Qi into the floor through the Bubbling Spring and also experiment with drawing Qi into the body through the same point from the floor.

Maintaining a good connection between Bubbling Spring and the floor is critical within our training. This is why it is so important that a Cat stance maintains contact between the ball of the foot on the front foot and the floor. We should feel 'grounded' through the Bubbling Spring point of both feet, no matter how our weight is distributed.

When Tai Chi teachers talk about full and empty legs or feet, you should consider whether they are talking about weight distribution or a more subtle aspect involving Qi flow into and/or out of the body through Bubbling Spring. Is a 'full' leg a leg where the flow of Qi is predominately inwards through Bubbling Spring or is it a leg where the Qi is flowing strongly down and out of Bubbling Spring? As always, with Tai Chi and Qigong it is often interpreting the words that are used that can be half the challenge! I would recommend experimenting by standing and stepping in different stances whilst trying different combinations of inwards and outwards flows – asking a partner to gently push you from different directions will help you to assess your grounded-ness (and relaxation!).

Within Tai Chi and Qigong training for health, our grounded-ness is important for our physical, mental and emotional health. Never underestimate the impact that the ways you use your physical body can have on your emotional and mental state. From a Chinese Medical perspective good health implies good physical, mental and emotional health.

If you find the one-legged stances difficult within your Tai Chi Forms or Qigong exercises you should spend time looking at how you are grounding. Consider the physical aspects of the stance first – are the joints correctly aligned? Are you too high (or low) in the stance? Is the standing foot aligned correctly? Are the muscles as relaxed as they should be? Make adjustments to experiment and find the best way to do each stance. Then consider the more subtle aspects – the Heel Vessels, Bubbling Spring, the Channels through the legs. Also, consider how you are feeling emotionally or mentally as these will affect your physical body just as much as the physical body will affect them.

Obviously, for the martial student grounding becomes another key aspect of Tai Chi Ch'uan training and Push Hands and similar exercises are essential methods for testing and improving grounding for martial purposes.

Chapter Thirteen.

Critical Distance.

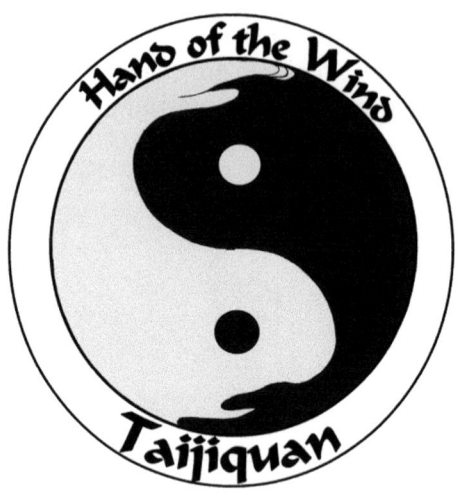

In Tai Chi we use the term 'critical distance' to describe the minimum amount of space that there should always be between the hand and the body. In simple terms, the hand should always be a full handspan (around eight inches or so) from the body. This means that the elbow also needs to be away from the body and a fist's width is the usual guide for the distance between elbow and body. It is also important for the arm to keep space from the body at the armpit and it is usually stated that there should be space for an 'egg' to be held within the armpit itself.

The reasons for always keeping this space between the body and the hand are twofold, firstly in martial terms the distance is necessary to prevent your limb getting trapped and either hitting yourself or allowing your opponent to gain control over your body; secondly, if the hand is too close to the body it introduces tension into various muscle groups in the body which will also restrict the flow of Qi.

For the hand to be closer to the upper body than the critical distance requires the elbow to bend to a sharper angle than ninety degrees and we have already stated in chapter nine that this should not be allowed to happen. Keeping the space in the armpit also keeps the area around the start of the Heart Channel (Heart acupoint number One) relaxed and therefore helps us to prevent ourselves becoming 'closed off'.

Use Standing Qigong practice to experiment with slight adjustments to the distance between the hand and the body – feel the quality of connection when lining up points in the hands with those in the body as a method for gauging good separation distances. Consider adjusting the position of the elbow as a way of reducing tension in the shoulders and arms as you adjust these distances. Often people hold the elbows too low or too tight to the body which builds tension into the chest as well as the shoulders.

While on the subject of elbows, it is another so-called 'rule' of Tai Chi that the elbows should be below the shoulders and when the hands are raised the elbow should sink below the wrist. There are clearly times within both our Tai Chi Form and within Qigong exercises where the elbow is above the shoulder – when arms are raised above head height for example. Care should be taken to consider whether this is achieved by opening the chest as discussed earlier or whether the arm is raised through the shoulder joint. When the arm is raised from the shoulder it is important to consider how you can maintain relaxation in the muscles around the shoulder and the back – experiment with the ways you can raise the arm by slightly adjusting the direction through which the arm raises.

When the hands are raised to around shoulder height, be careful to maintain the correct amount of bend in the elbow and to keep the shoulder relaxed – doing this will ensure that the elbow will be below the height of the shoulder and the wrist. Also, be aware of the angle of the hand – if the hand is raised to the side to shoulder height and the little finger edge is directed upward (with the palm facing away from the body) then the elbow will come too high. You need to adjust the hand to around a forty-five-degree angle and the elbow will lower to the correct position. Again, experiment with holding positions to feel where the tensions arise and then make adjustments to discover the most relaxed positions.

Chapter Fourteen.

The Centre Line.

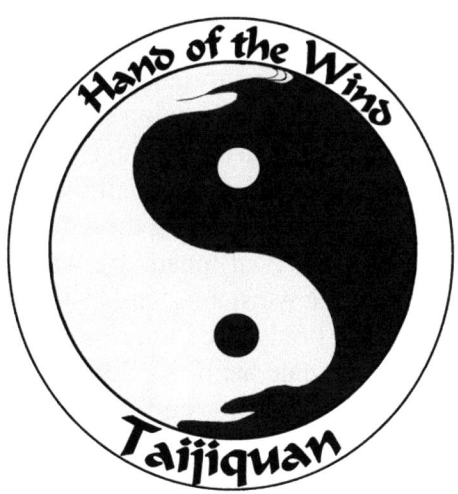

One of the often quoted 'rules' of Tai Chi Ch'uan is that the hand should never cross the centre line. There are two main issues with this rule which are evident even to beginners. One is that the hands sometimes cross past each other in our Tai Chi Form – try doing that without crossing the centre line! The other is that if I am blocking a punch coming towards the centre of my face then it is obvious that my hand is going to have to cross the centre line.

This 'rule' is, therefore, something which requires further investigation. If I were to move my hand across my chest without allowing the shoulders to be disrupted it clearly introduces tension in the pectoral muscles of the chest. This tension is apparent even if I maintain the critical distance between hand and body by adjusting elbow angles. We therefore require techniques which allow the hand to come past the centre without introducing these tensions.

There are two practical means by which I can achieve this – turning from the waist and 'collapsing' the chest. As a general guideline, if I only need to bring one hand across the centre line and the other hand is effectively passive at that point then I would turn from the waist. This is commonly seen in movements which derive from a simple ward-off and strike type movement – the turn of the waist allows us to block the incoming strike and provides us with 'coiled' power to then launch our own strike. A good example from the Lee Style Tai Chi Form would be movement number twenty-six.

As the waist turns be aware of the 'spiralling' feeling around the spine and consider how the Qi of the Thrusting and Belt Vessels is involved in the movement. It is important to ensure that the turn of the waist is as relaxed as possible but to not corrupt the stance by twisting the pelvis – do remember to keep the stance 'soft' and avoid tension, particularly around the gluteal muscles and the inguinal area.

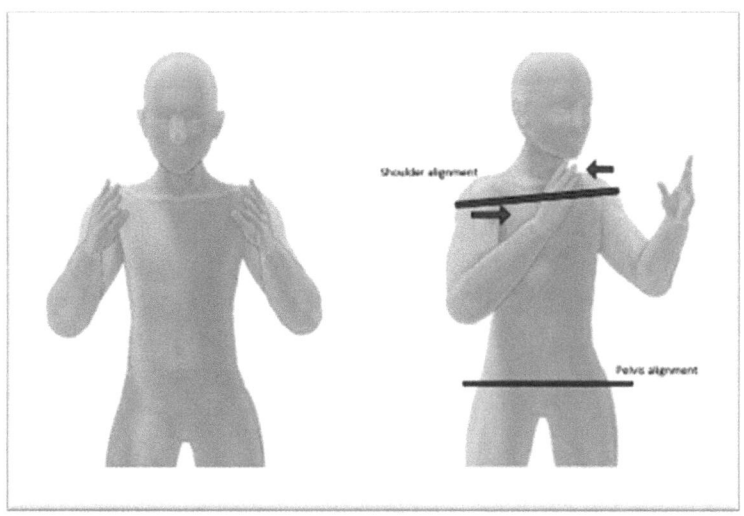

Fig. 34 Turning the Waist.

The other option is perhaps the more difficult of the two – the 'collapse' of the chest. To get the idea of this movement, bring one of your hands up to chest height in front of the body with the palm facing the shoulder (so lining up Lao Gong with Qi Hu), then allow the shoulder to roll inwards bringing the hand effectively across the chest. Make sure that you are not tightening the muscles across the chest to pull the hand across – the movement is more to do with relaxing the muscles between the shoulder blades and allowing the sternum at the centre of the chest to sink slightly. There is a very strong inward contraction or Yin feel within the chest and a strong expansion or Yang feel across the back. It feels almost as if you are allowing yourself to begin to curl up into a ball. Contrast this feeling with the expansion of the chest discussed in chapter nine in order to raise the arms above shoulder height.

This technique of 'collapsing' the chest is used when both arms apparently cross the centre line and is most evident in those movements where the arms actually cross past each other (as in movements twelve or seventeen of the Lee Family Tai Chi Form).

To complicate things even further, it is often necessary to combine both of these techniques into a single movement. This is seen in the Tai Chi Form in those movements where a hand passes the centre whilst the other hand is still 'active'. A good example would be in movement number thirty-three where the turn of the waist acts as an evasion from an incoming strike (guarded by the right hand) and both arms effectively cross the centre line at the same time.

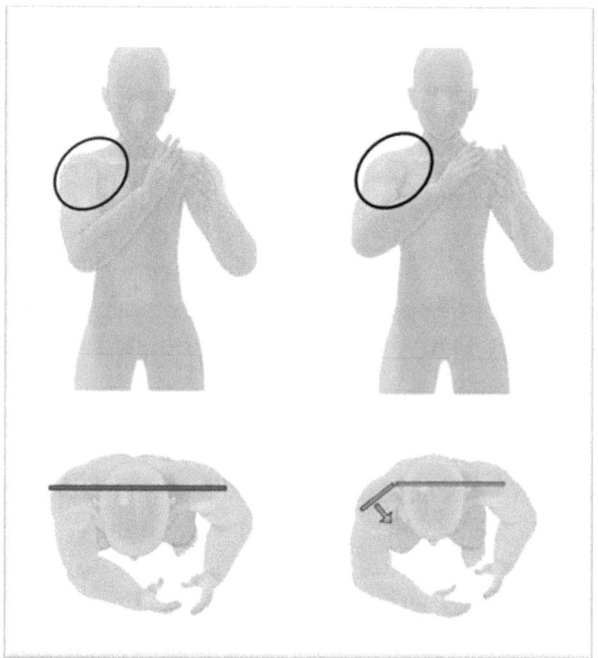

Fig. 35 Collapsing the Shoulder.

Chapter Fifteen.

Relaxation.

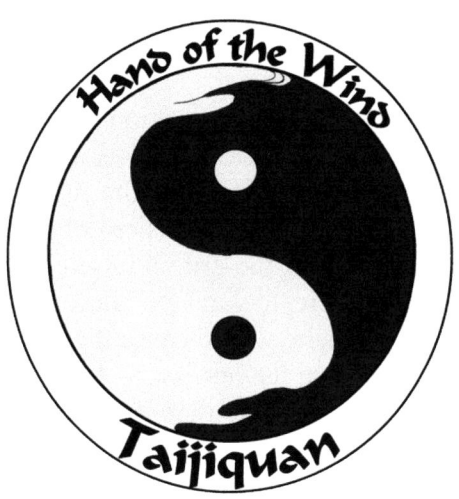

Throughout this text you will have noticed that relaxation is something that we constantly come back to when talking about Tai Chi and Qigong. In order for the body to function at its best we need to ensure that it is not over-working and that Qi is allowed to flow smoothly throughout the body. To do this, we need to make sure that there is no excess tension within the body.

Within our training we strive to always be as relaxed as possible and then to carry that into all other aspects of our lives. The key point in the previous sentence is 'as possible' – if we were completely relaxed, we would be lying on the floor unable to move!

To explain the level of relaxation required, we often use the phrase 'dynamic tension'. This means the absolute minimum amount of tension that the muscles of the body require in order to achieve the desired objective. The usual example given is that if the arm is raised to shoulder height and a snowflake were to land on the arm, then the extra weight of the snowflake would cause the arm to lower.

So, some tension is necessary to simply maintain a posture but it is important that there is no extra tension anywhere in the body. Most people constantly carry excess tension throughout their bodies and in fact, some muscles of their bodies are actively 'fighting' against each other all of the time. If we can eliminate this excess tension so that our bodies are working as one unit rather than continuing these internal struggles then our bodies are less likely to wear themselves out – this is one of the key ways in which Tai Chi and Qigong can help us to maintain good levels of health.

In order to reduce the levels of tension that we carry within our bodies we firstly need to become more aware of our own bodies and to actually feel the tensions within the muscles. Regular effective Tai Chi and Qigong practice will greatly increase your ability to be aware of these tensions and then this will allow you to gradually release them.

It could be considered that Tai Chi is the easiest thing in the World because all you have to do is move naturally and without excess effort! The reality is, of course, that we have spent many years building up tensions within our bodies (physically, mentally and emotionally) and it does take time to release them. Do not expect to master relaxation as soon as you start training Tai Chi and Qigong – it will take time! The good thing is that, from the first time you start to practice, you will start to release some of these tensions and it then becomes an ongoing process that will continue to yield benefits for many years to come.

Holding a posture (whether when doing Standing Qigong or just pausing at the end point of a movement in the Tai Chi Form) is a good way to become more aware of the tensions in your body. When you hold a posture, after a while you will notice muscles which start to ache – these muscles are therefore working hard and you should try to relax them. Make small, subtle adjustments to the posture to find more relaxed ways of holding the body in position. Practicing movements as slowly as you can will give you the time to notice and release tensions. This is why Tai Chi Forms and Qigong exercises should be performed slowly – to enable the maximum amount of relaxation. For the Qigong breathing exercises, aim to time the movement to the breath and to slow the breaths down over time.

A classic phrase often associated with Tai Chi is 'to use four ounces to move a thousand pounds.' This gives us a clear indication of the idea of using minimum tension or force to achieve the desired outcome. In a purely physical sense, it also indicates how important timing and angles are when considering movements and postures. Again, this is particularly important for students of the martial aspects of Tai Chi Ch'uan.

Chapter Sixteen.

Breathing.

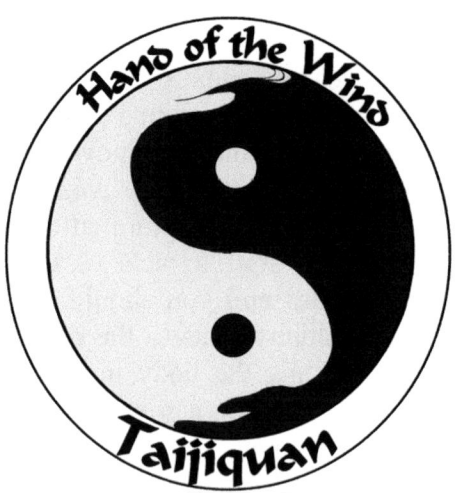

When considering the practice of Tai Chi and Qigong, breathing is central to everything that we do. Breathing should be naturally deep and relaxed. As mentioned previously, the literal translation of Qi is usually given as 'breath' and most systems of health Qigong consist of sets of breathing exercises where movements and breathing are harmonized.

Within our Lee Family Style Tai Chi Form training, it is important not to try to force the breathing to work with the Form too early. Beginning students often ask whether they should be breathing in or out in a particular movement of the Form and my answer is always 'don't worry about it!' If you try to make the breathing and movements linked, all you will do is build tension into your Tai Chi Form. You will either get stressed because you feel you are doing it 'wrong' or you will end up rushing a movement so as not to run out of breath. Alternatively, you will rush the breath to fit the movement or, even worse, end up holding your breath waiting for the next movement to start.

If you practice your Tai Chi effectively, use breathing exercises to work on your breathing and build the relaxation into your body, then over time the breathing will naturally harmonize with the Tai Chi Form movements – probably without you even realising it. Give it time!

In order to improve the quality of your breathing there are two main ways that we train breathing within our Tai Chi and Qigong. The first method is called 'Three Store Breathing' and is a way of encouraging people to breathe more deeply and use more of their lung capacity. It is a somewhat 'tense' method of training breathing as it uses the muscles of the body to work the lungs.

To practice 'Three Store Breathing', think of the body as divided into three sections; the lower 'store' is the abdomen from the navel downwards, the middle 'store' covers the area from the navel up to the bottom of the sternum (breastbone) and the 'upper' store covers the chest (the area enclosed by the ribcage).

When breathing in, aim to fill the lower store first so as the breath fills the lungs the diaphragm pushes down onto the abdominal organs and pushes the lower abdomen out forwards. Then, fill the middle store by allowing the upper part of the abdomen to also become extended. Once the middle store is filled, then allow the chest to expand as the lungs fully expand. During the out-breath this order is reversed, so that you empty the upper store first, then the middle and then the lower.

To help get the hang of this 'Three Store Breathing', place one hand on your abdomen below the navel and the other above the navel. Whilst breathing out, press inwards with the top hand first and then the lower. As you breathe in, keep the pressure on the abdomen with the top hand and allow the breath to push the lower hand outwards. Then reduce the pressure on the top hand to allow the middle store to fill, before filling the upper store. This can also be done as a partner exercise, by lying on the floor (on your back – supine) and having a partner sit or kneel next to you and place their hands onto your abdomen (one above and one below the navel). Your partner can then adjust the pressure on each of their hands to help you feel and control the breath into each of the three stores.

'Three Store Breathing' is a good exercise for getting people to breathe more deeply and to encourage people to use their diaphragm more effectively within the breath – so it is particularly useful for people who breathe more in their chests without the abdomen expanding. I have noticed over the years that I have been teaching these arts that fewer students seem to come into the classes who are just breathing in the chest – perhaps due to the increase in popularity of yoga, Pilates and singing. It has, however, become noticeable that more people are not using the intercostal muscles and the ribcage as effectively within their breathing now though!

For breathing to be truly effective there should be both the characteristic movement of the abdomen related to deep breathing and the expansion and contraction of the chest as the ribs are lifted and separated during the in-breath and then drawn back down in the out-breath.

This brings us to the second method of training breathing – the relaxed breath method. This can be done standing, seated or lying – as long as the body is relaxed. First, focus on your natural breathing and allow yourself to be aware of how the body moves with the breath. Concentrate on the in-breath and feel how deep into the chest your breath 'reaches'. Then, be aware of the muscles in the chest and abdomen and how they are working with the breath – notice the tensions. Start to work on bringing the breath deeper into the chest – just slightly with each in-breath. Do this by breathing in until you feel the first signs of tension within the torso – as soon as you feel any tension allow the breath to exit the body. With practice you will be able to sink the breath further and further down into the body before you start to tense up the muscles.

Both of these methods are intended to encourage students of Tai Chi and Qigong to breathe more deeply and use more of their lung capacity. Most people use only a small proportion of the capacity of their lungs when breathing normally. By breathing more deeply, you will introduce more oxygen into your body and expel more carbon dioxide from the body. Often beginning students find that they can feel light-headed when practicing Tai Chi or Qigong (particularly when focusing on their breathing a lot) until the body adjusts to breathing more deeply.

Practice both methods of increasing lung capacity and aim to become more aware of your breathing in everyday life. As you practice Qigong breathing exercises, work on slowing the breath and the movement and be aware of the interaction between the movement and the breath. Notice how the expansion and contraction of the breath corresponds with expansions and contractions within the movements.

Chapter Seventeen.

The Eight Energies.

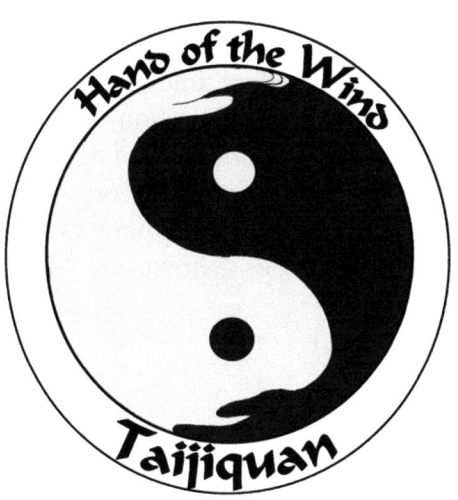

In its simplest terms Tai Chi Ch'uan can be said to be practicing the 'Eight Energies' in the 'Five Directions'. This covers all the complexities of the movements within the Tai Chi Forms as the Eight Energies teach how the body moves within each posture of the Form. The Eight Energies are often emphasized more by the martial students of Tai Chi but it is essential to gain a measure of understanding of them in order to perform the Tai Chi Forms correctly and therefore gain the maximum health benefits.

The 'Five Directions' do not require much explanation as they are simply: to the front, to the rear, to each side and staying in the centre. Sometimes, teachers of Tai Chi and Qigong say that these five directions each correspond with one of the Five Transformations but I personally feel that the explanations for these particular correspondences always seem somewhat forced and are actually unnecessary.

The Eight Energies, however, do require some explanation.

The Eight Energies are:

Ward Off – 'Peng'
Roll Back – 'Lu'
Push – 'An'
Press Down– 'Ji'

Squeeze/Grasp/Press – 'Tsai'
Split/Rend – 'Lieh'
Elbow – 'Chou'
Shoulder – 'Kao'

The first four are considered the 'primary' set of Energies and the others are considered 'secondary'. Each of these 'Energies' informs our movements both on a physical level and a more subtle Qi based level. In order to master them it is necessary to first consider and feel them on a physical, more external, level before internalizing them and moving on to the more subtle levels. Probably, the biggest mistake any student of Tai Chi can make is to try to master the subtle levels before understanding the physical.

We shall look at each of the Eight Energies in turn and examine how physical movements can help us to understand them. Internalizing the Eight Energies requires good levels of relaxation throughout the body and a high level of Qi sensitivity – and therefore takes time!

Peng or Ward Off

Peng (pronounced more like 'pung') is usually the first of the Eight Energies that students of Hand of the Wind Taijiquan will be taught. There are numerous partner exercises commonly taught within the Lee Family Arts that can help with gaining an understanding of Peng including Two Hands Against Two, Two Hands Against One and of course Push Hands.

If you bring your arm up to chest height and ask a partner to press your arm towards your body, Peng is the means by which we aim to prevent our arm collapsing back against the body – it 'wards off' the press from the other person. The key thing to consider and work on is to make this as relaxed as possible. Experiment with different angles of the elbow and wrist, be aware of the shoulder and the back to avoid tension. For the person pressing on to your arm the feeling that they should get is often described as a 'resilience'. It should not feel hard or rigid - but should have a softness present along with the feel that the arm is not going to collapse to the body.

As more pressure is applied to the arm, it is important that we do not tense up and become rigid – there will come a point where the press will overcome the Peng! It is also important that, if the press is suddenly removed from our arm, then our arm does not 'spring' away from the body indicating that we are using tension to push the other person away.

The 'energy' (or perhaps 'feeling' would be a better word) of Peng is vital for maintaining our critical distance and not allowing the hand or elbow to get too close to the body. Use partner exercises to get the feel of Peng and then work on maintaining the same feeling within the body even when there is no external pressure being applied. This then allows you to start to internalize the feeling – just always remember to relax and then relax some more! You can feel the quality of the energy just by placing your hand onto the arm of someone who is skilled in the use of Peng – it will feel alive and dynamic; very soft with a core of strength lying beneath.

Lu or Roll Back

When our partner presses on to our arm, as described above in the section on Peng, there comes a point where the push will overcome the Peng or tension takes over (note that the more skilled the practitioner, then the 'stronger' the Peng will be and will therefore resist greater pressures).

When our bodies are placed under excess pressure, the energy of Lu comes into play. Lu is sometimes described as the defining energy of Tai Chi Ch'uan but without Peng it becomes meaningless.

Consider the beginning of a game of single-handed push hands as shown in the following diagrams. Both 'players' set up with their arms touching and each having a feeling of Peng. Person A then presses forwards on the arm of Person B by advancing forwards in their stance. Person B feels that their Peng is going to be overcome (staying relaxed and warding off the entire body weight of another person is not easy!), so Person B yields. This yielding as they move

106

backwards in their stance combined with the turning of the waist to redirect Person A's push is a simple physical manifestation of the energy (or feeling) of Lu.*Fig.*

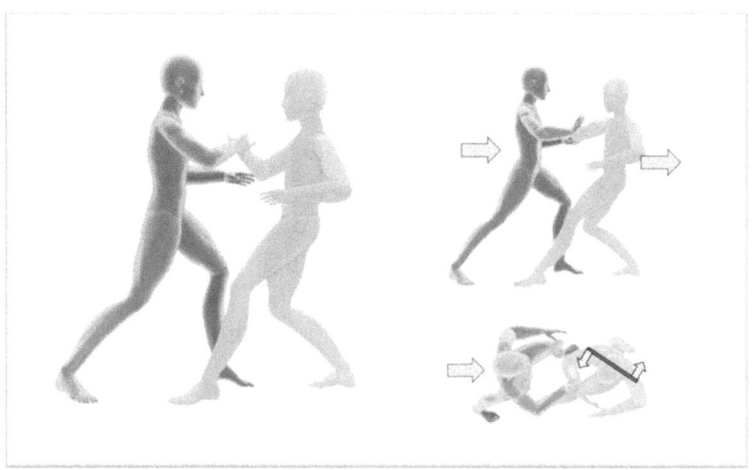

36 Feeling Lu 'Energy' with a partner.

Note that throughout this 'yielding' process, Person B maintains their Peng so that their arm is not pressed back against their body.

Lu is usually described as 'roll back' by most instructors of Tai Chi as the term 'yield' does not suggest the idea of the turning quality which is an essential part of Lu. Lu does not mean to simply give way to a force, it implies the redirection of the incoming force to prevent it becoming a problem. This is usually achieved through the turning of the waist as shown in the diagram – but it is a worthwhile exercise to thoroughly explore other ways in which the same feeling of redirecting an incoming force can be achieved whilst maintaining relaxation and Peng – Lu is not just in the horizontal plane! Again, this kind of exploration of Lu and Peng forms a major part of the training for students of the martial aspects of Tai Chi Ch'uan.

An or Push

To push within the martial context of Tai Chi Ch'uan also covers to strike or kick – whilst maintaining relaxation. Be aware of the spine and the co-ordination of the pelvis and shoulders whenever you execute a push type movement – you should feel the way the torso opens or expands in the direction of the push which is a characteristic aspect of An. Within the Tai Chi Form there are numerous An or Push type movements utilizing the arms and sometimes they are performed with more of an 'over-arm' type of movement and sometimes with more of an 'under-arm' type movement. This affects the way that the pelvis and shoulders interact and therefore how the spine moves within the movement.

The power of a Push comes from the floor, via the legs and is controlled from the centre of the body. It is not just a matter of pushing the hand forwards with the muscles of the arm and shoulder! The true strength of An comes from the whole body moving as a unit in the direction of the Push.

Much has been made of the so-called 'elastic' force of Tai Chi Ch'uan and this is usually demonstrated in a Push Hands type context where one person pushes forwards onto the demonstrator, who then yields (Lu) whilst maintaining their Peng before allowing the body to unwind back towards the 'attacker' using the feeling of An. This recoil to spring requires relaxation through the body and correct alignment of the body with particular attention paid to the pelvis, spine and shoulders.

From a health perspective the quality of An that is most desirable is the connection throughout a relaxed body and the loosening and opening of the spine. It is very important to relax the muscles of the back in order to prevent the individual vertebrae of the spine from being compressed towards each other. This can then allow the flexibility within the spine which is necessary for An. Within Chinese Internal

108

martial arts, loosening of the spine is required to enable the 'whip' of the spine which is used in hand strikes (and which is a form of An or Push). But, again from a health perspective, it is the co-ordination of hips/pelvis and shoulders and how they are connected by the spine which needs to be concentrated upon as it is not necessary to practice the 'whip' of the spine with the same level of explosive effect that is required by the martial students.

Ji or Press Down

The last of the four primary 'Energies' is Ji or Press Down. This is often viewed as the pressing down with the hand but this is just one of the physical manifestations of Ji. Within the Shou Pai Fa Form usually taught within the Lee Family system of Feng Shou Kung Fu, the opening movements give a good simple demonstration of Lu, followed by Ji and then a move into An. This can be practiced easily with a partner by starting in the usual single-handed Push Hands opening position. As person A presses forwards and person B 'rolls back' (Lu), then person B lays the palm of their hand (the same hand that is already in contact!) onto the top of person A's arm and presses down until in front of their hip, the palm then turns towards person A and pushes forwards towards their chest. This is also one of the movements that can be used to transfer from a horizontal circle to the vertical circle when practicing single-handed Push Hands.

Whilst this press down using the hand is a clear and useful example of Ji, it can cause problems with students who then view Ji as just pressing down with the hand. As always with Tai Chi and Qigong, we need to look at what is happening within the body during the movement - so what happens in the body that allows the arm to press downwards?

Make sure that you are not using tension to push their arm downwards, the feeling should come from within the body. Look for the muscle changes within the body and then over time, feel how the Qi moves within the body during the movement of the arm. You can then start to see how the energy or feeling of Ji can be used in other movements – not just pressing downwards with the hand or arm.

This process of learning the physical, external movement and then looking deeper and deeper inwards to find the subtle 'energetic' movement of Qi is how Tai Chi changes from a physical exercise to a more holistic pursuit involving the body, the mind and the more subtle flows of Qi.

The four primary 'Energies' of Tai Chi discussed so far, often are as far as many students really explore within the Tai Chi. They do, after all, incorporate feelings of expansion and contraction throughout the body and therefore bring the concepts of Yin and Yang into our practice. Even amongst Tai Chi practitioners who incorporate regular Pushing Hands practice into their training, they often don't really progress beyond an understanding of Peng, Lu, Ji and An. This is not intended as a criticism – it is merely an acknowledgement of the depth and utility of the four primary Energies which means that a practitioner can be effective without pushing themselves to look deeper.

Part of the beauty of Tai Chi is that there are great depths available to those students that wish to explore further – and that great benefits can be obtained without necessarily needing to devote the time required to achieve such a full understanding of all aspects of the art.

To continue with our exploration of the Eight Energies we will now examine the 'secondary' Energies of Tsai, Lieh, Chou and Kao. Remember, when thinking about the Eight Energies, first examine the physical and then look deeper into yourself to find the subtleties of each of them and how they are utilized within each. The descriptions of the secondary Energies presented here are very brief as it is very difficult to explain the feelings in simple text – the input of an instructor in person and hands on training is necessary to really gain an understanding of these Energies.

Tsai or Squeeze

This is another of the Eight Energies which is often described in quite varied ways. It is sometimes described as a 'Grasp' or a 'Pluck', sometimes as 'Press' but within Hand of the Wind classes we usually use the term 'Squeeze'. A physical movement which is often used as an example of Tsai is when a fist closes as if 'grasping' such as in movement number twenty-one of the Lee Family Tai Chi Form. However, this can again lead to students thinking that it is about the hand and not about what is happening in the body.

If you really examine the movement of move number twenty-one, you can feel muscle changes within the chest as the hand 'grasps' – it can be useful to exaggerate the closing of the fist to accentuate the movements within the body. It is this feeling within the body that we call Tsai – not the closing of the hand. Once you feel how the body effects the closing of the hand, you can then start to see how this 'squeeze' within the body is also used within other movements.

Again, work from the physical inwards by following the muscle changes and then build on your sensitivity to make your Tai Chi more subtle and therefore Internal.

Lieh or Rend

Lieh is characterized by a rending or splitting movement so is often seen in movements where the arms move away from each other in opposite directions. Again, examine the movement in more detail and you will start to feel how the movement originates from the centre and is controlled through the body. Lieh also incorporates movements where the upper and lower bodies move in seemingly opposite directions and like Tsai is therefore involved in turning the waist.

If we consider the chest, we can see that in a Lieh type movement the chest is usually opening or expanding and this feels almost like the opposite of a Tsai feeling where the chest feels as if it is compressing more. Consider the Yin and Yang of both of these movements (think about front and back of the body, upper and lower body, etc.) and also explore how the vertical and horizontal components interact with each other.

Chou or Elbow

The last two of the Eight Energies can be even more difficult for students to isolate from the physical action – particularly as they are usually referred to as 'Elbow' and 'Shoulder'. From a simple martial perspective Chou does indeed include the physical actions of striking with the elbow – but again it is necessary to look deeper.

Consider the angles at which an elbow can lead a movement (inward, outward, upward, downward) and it is clear that they can all be used as effective striking techniques with the elbow as the weapon. But when you look further into the muscle changes that drive the elbow in each of these angles, you can start to find some common ground that they all share. It is then necessary to consider those muscle changes and movements deeper within the body without the context of the elbow at all. This then leads to an understanding of the feeling of Chou and how it does not always, in fact, incorporate a strike with the elbow.

For the student of Tai Chi and Qigong for Health, being able to execute an effective elbow strike really is not important. It is important, however, to understand the way the body moves and releases the flow of Qi within Chou influenced movements.

Do remember, when examining how Chou is manifested throughout the body that the stance is still part of the movement. Often people can get too fixated on the upper body and can forget that the driving force for everything in Tai Chi comes from the legs. We must always strive to maintain the harmony between stance and posture if we want our bodies to work in a truly relaxed manner.

Kao or Shoulder

Sometimes referred to as 'bump', Kao is demonstrated when we use our shoulder to impact an opponent in the martial application of Tai Chi Ch'uan. It is important to look at how the whole body is incorporated within this simple application and to feel how muscle changes through the body allow the shoulder to lead in the desired direction. As with Chou, the correct use of stance is critical in understanding Kao and to understand that the 'energy' of Kao does not require the shoulder to be used to strike a target at all.

As an interesting example, try to feel the muscle changes within the body in movement number thirty-four of the Lee Style Tai Chi Form as the shoulder leads the forwards movement. Then, compare those muscle changes with the ones required in order to bring the leg around in movement number thirty-eight.

It is by looking for similarities between different movements that, at first glance, look to be very different that we start to understand the complexities of the interactions between the Eight Energies and their application in each of the Five Directions.

No single movement of Tai Chi Form (or indeed any movement within a Qigong exercise) will simply use one of the Eight Energies – every movement incorporates some aspect of all of them. This is why it is often said that every movement of the Tai Chi Form hides a strike, a kick, a parry, a lock, a throw, etc.

By considering the interactions between the Eight Energies on a subtle level we can start to understand how the flow of Qi through our bodies affects (and effects) our movements. This can then, in turn, lead us to more relaxed, more powerful movements which can help to keep our bodies functioning in the way they naturally should in accordance with the Tao.

Appendix.

Quick Reference Guide.

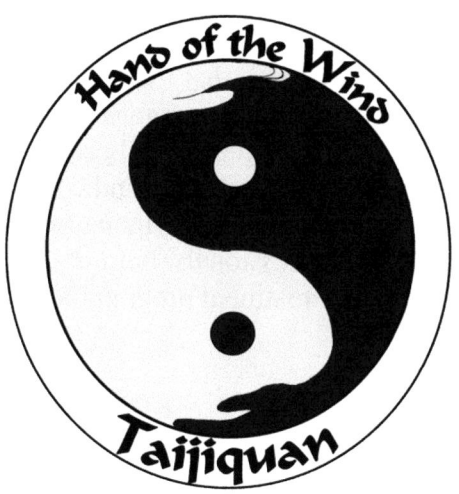

Within this appendix you will find a quick reference guide to each of the Five Transformations outlining their Channels, Gates, associations and pointers towards relevant Qigong exercises.

The specific named Taoyin Qigong exercises are chosen from the most commonly practiced exercises within Hand of the Wind Taijiquan classes and should be familiar to most practitioners of the Lee Family Internal Arts. These are just examples of exercises that would be beneficial for each of the Five Transformations and are by no means an exhaustive list. The examples are simply intended to give students a feel for the types of exercises that are beneficial for each transformation. Each of the examples given are outlined in the Hand of the Wind Taijiquan publication, Taoyin Qigong, available through www.handofthewind.co.uk.

It is vital that any student of Qigong seeks guidance from suitably qualified professionals before using any Qigong exercises as part of a treatment programme for any diagnosed ailment

I
Fire

Yin Channel:	**Heart** **Heart Protector**
Yang Channel:	**Small Intestine** **Triple Heater**
Channel Location:	**Little finger edge of arm (HT/SI).** **Centre of underside and back of arm (HP/TH).**
Gate:	**Laogong (HP)** **Yang Gu (SI)**
Emotion:	**Joy**
Sense Organ:	**Tongue**
Tissue:	**Blood Vessels**
Associations:	**Emotional associations with heart, including receptivity and emotional open-ness. Communication and speech. Temperature regulation and control of 'fluids' in the body.**
Movement in Qigong:	**Arms raised to front or above head.**
Taoyin Exercises	**Support the Clouds.** **Separate the Clouds.** **Happy Day.**

II
Earth

Yin Channel:	**Spleen**
Yang Channel:	**Stomach**
Channel Location:	**Front and sides of body, front of legs.**
Gate:	**Qi Hu**
Emotion:	**Sympathy**
Sense Organ:	**Lips**
Tissue:	**Muscles**
Associations:	**Digestion of food and ideas. Thinking and overthinking. Muscles and regulation of blood.**
Movement in Qigong:	**Stretching of the sides and front of body by twisting or leaning. Stretches of the front of the legs.**
Taoyin Exercises:	**Move the Rainbow. Play the Shuttlecock. Bend and Twist.**

III
Metal

Yin Channel:	**Lung**
Yang Channel:	**Large Intestine**
Channel Location:	**Thumb 'edge' of arm.**
Gate:	**He Gu**
Emotion:	**Grief**
Sense Organ:	**Nose**
Tissue:	**Skin**
Associations:	**Breathing, connection between the internal and external.** **The skin and touch.** **Ability to 'let things go'.**
Movement in Qigong:	**Arms raised to sides.**
Taoyin Exercises:	**Archer Turns Around.** **Expand the Chest.** **The Flying Fox.**

IV
Water

Yin Channel:	**Kidney**
Yang Channel:	**Bladder**
Channel Location:	**Back of legs and body.**
Gate:	**Yong Quan**
Emotion:	**Fear**
Sense Organ:	**Ears**
Tissue:	**Bones**
Associations:	**Vitality, creativity, courage. Bones and nervous system. Ears and hearing.**
Movement in Qigong:	**Leaning forwards or backwards. Stretches of hamstrings and the back of the legs.**
Taoyin:	**The Moving Mirror. Bend and Twist. The Growing Pine.**

V
Tree

Yin Channel:	**Liver**
Yang Channel:	**Gall Bladder**
Channel Location:	**Sides of body and head. Centre of the inside and outside of the legs.**
Gate:	**Huan Tsai**
Emotion:	**Anger**
Sense Organ:	**Eyes**
Tissue:	**Tendons**
Associations:	**Flexibility and adaptability. Planning ahead and moving forwards (and upwards). Joints and tendons. Eyes and eyesight.**
Movement in Qigong:	**Stretching the sides of the body thorough leaning or twisting.**
Taoyin:	**The Dragon Spits Fire. Rotate the Wheel. Step Forwards and Look Back.**

Afterword:
A comment from the author.

I have been training in these arts for over a quarter of a century now and I am aware that the way I practice and teach the arts has changed enormously over the years. However, I have always believed that people perform better when they understand what they are trying to achieve and this book is aimed at making that easier for students of Hand of the Wind Taijiquan.

This volume contains much of the theory that I try to convey to my students within classes. In parts this is deliberately simplified – most students do not need or desire to learn every aspect of Traditional Chinese Medicine in order to improve their health using Tai Chi and Qigong. Some things are very hard to explain in print (the Eight Energies!) and some aspects of Tai Chi and Qigong do just need to be learnt (point locations for the 'Gates').

It is my hope that this book will help you, the reader, to gain at least some small measure of understanding of the theory behind your practice and that this will help you to gain more benefits and more enjoyment from that practice. Hopefully this book raises questions, as well as answering a few at least. A questioning attitude towards your training will encourage you to look ever deeper into your Tai Chi and Qigong – and that is a good thing!

As always, enjoy your training and I hope you continue to enjoy the benefits for many years to come.

Conrad Robinson 2020.

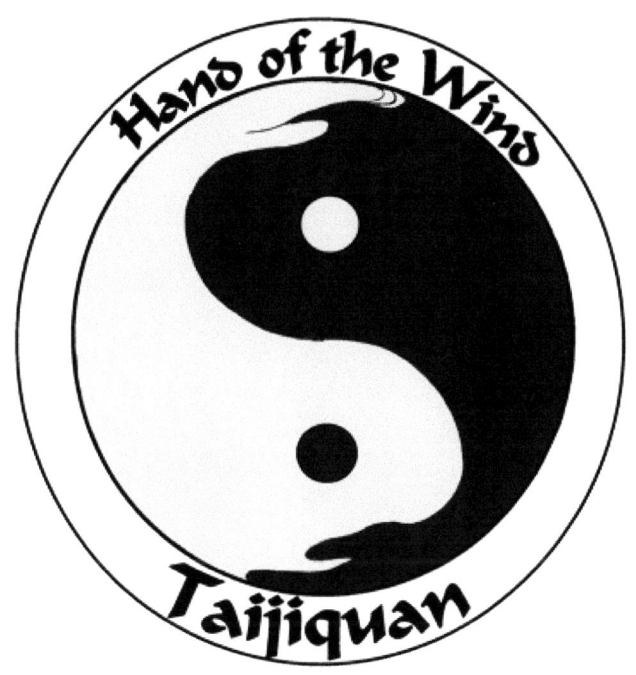

Notes:

Notes:

Notes